COUNTRY DOCTOR

Tales of a rural GP

COUNTRY DOCTOR

Tales of a rural GP

Dr Michael Sparrow

ROBINSON
London

Constable & Robinson Ltd
3 The Lanchesters
162 Fulham Palace Road
London W6 9ER
www.constablerobinson.com

First published in the UK by Robinson,
an imprint of Constable & Robinson Ltd, 2002

A copy of the British Library Cataloguing in
Publication Data is available from the British Library.

ISBN 1-84119-421-2

Printed and bound in the EU

10 9 8 7 6 5 4 3 2 1

For my children, Charlie and Cressie, and in memory of my mother, Mary Blackmore, née Hopkins, who died after a short illness on 5 August 2001, several months prior to publication.

She did, however, manage to read a copy of both this and the draft of the next book in the last week of her life. 'Oh,' she said as she put it down for the final time. 'So that's what you've been doing for the past twenty-five years . . .'

Acknowledgements

The author wishes to thank all those who have helped – unwittingly or otherwise – and encouraged during the production of this book, but a special note of thanks to Lorna Hartley, who typed the very first draft and without whom this would still be sitting at the back of some dusty cupboard written on odd scraps of paper. So for all of you who do not enjoy what you are about to read – it's her fault.

Contents

Introduction

A couple of years ago, one of the august weekly medical journals for GPs – we refer to them reverentially as 'the comics' – ran a writing competition under the heading 'What advice would you give to prospective GPs?'

I have no idea what they expected – carefully researched tributes to the exquisite delights and vocational rewards of our chosen profession, perhaps?

What they got was something rather different.

One entrant, for example – who failed to secure one of the ten winners' slots but was unanimously voted for a life peerage by us all – simply wrote, 'Don't do it, don't do it, don't do it . . .' two hundred times, and we all knew how he felt.

Collectively we advanced enough reasons to avoid the job to put off a whole generation of putative doctors for life. Our entries remain locked in an underground vault, to be published posthumously.

The ten winners were invited to a weekend jamboree in Tunbridge Wells, where we soberly assessed the thrills of our profession, the sheer unadulterated pleasure of spending our days face to face with the collective woes of the general public, and the craftsmanship of writing. It took all of five minutes, and then we repaired to the bar, this particular discussion being over for the night.

What now follows is an amended version of what I then wrote, which along with the other nine entries should be force-fed to all sixth-formers as they consider their future career prospects.

Beyond that, a collection of anecdotes from now some twenty years in medicine, neither wholly autobiographical nor terribly chronological, but more like a busy morning surgery the day after a bank holiday.

It is the one everlasting joy of general practice. You never quite know what is going to walk through the door next.

To a Prospective GP . . .

Dear son,

I know you are considering taking up general practice as a career. May I give you some advice.

1. Watch every episode of *Peak Practice*, twice – it's brilliant. Marvel at their dedication. Thrill to their diagnostic skills. Rejoice at their successes and empathise with their tragedies. Wonder how come they only ever see one patient per week. Count how many times Andrew smiles during any one episode. And then disregard everything you see. It's just not like that at all.

2. Get yourself fit. I suggest running up a down escalator for ten hours a day. Capture that feeling at the end of each session, and remember it well. We call it exhaustion, and it will stay with you for the rest of your career.

3. Enroll with RADA. It will help you cultivate that expression of concerned professionalism, behind which are your true thoughts – 'If I can dispense with Mrs Pemberton's leg ulcers in the next five minutes, I can still get in nine holes of golf before lunch.'

4. Get yourself a very large mirror. Practise before it for six hours a day until you can say, 'It's only a virus,' and 'I know how you feel,' not to mention 'There's a lot of it about,' without giggling helplessly.

5. Spend as much time as you can with a circus. Run away with

2

it if possible, but if not, then study the man who balances twenty spinning plates on long poles (do not be put off by the fact that you recognise him as being also the Lithuanian tight-rope walker). Note how he always attends to the most needy first. And before you leave, enter the cage full of lions. It's not quite so bad as a packed waiting room on a rainy Monday morning, but boy, is it close.

6. Start smoking, and persevere. Then no matter how bad it may get, you will still be able to enjoy yourself up to twenty times a day.

7. Practise self-catheterisation, and subscribe to a 'Teach Yourself Colonic Irrigation' course. Only then will you understand what it can be like to deal with health service administrators.

8. Develop a liking for Lambrusco and cheap whisky. I know it will be hard, but it is all your patients will ever buy you for Christmas.

9. Let every meal you sit down to go cold, and stodgy. Ask a close friend to bleep you every time you get into a hot bath, or when England look poised to win at anything, and learn to cope with the inevitable frustration that will follow.

10. Invest in the Which? guide to divorce. Do not be deterred by the fact that you are not yet married – you will be, and then you will not.

11. Read all the political columns of the broadsheet newspapers. Become a doctor of spin, as well as of medicine.

12. Purchase the most uncomfortable bed on the market. That way, you will never mind leaving it on a cold winter's morning.

These are the twelve commandments. As my old Latin master used to say – learn, inwardly digest, and repeat at will.

And should all else fail, just study your father. Observe his stress-free countenance. Rejoice at his new-found joie de vivre, marvel at his careless good humour.

Recall that you have only seen him thus since he took early retirement. Recall, in fact, that you have scarcely seen him at all before that fateful day, and that one day you too will have children.

Ask yourself – is that what you really want?

And finally, we will one day meet at one of our funerals. I pray that it is mine. And not yours . . .

All this, of course, is now incidental for the likes of me. Twenty years qualified and beyond the realms of reason, no longer do we ask ourselves why we became a GP, but only why we still are one.

And I have two answers:

1. Because I am no longer trained for, or capable of doing, anything else.
2. And because if I wasn't a GP, then none of the following would have happened.

And somehow – I would have missed it.

1

Doomed from the Start

It isn't easy, travelling through life with a surname like Sparrow. All those 'Tweet tweet, dicky bird' jokes wear a bit thin after the first couple of thousand outings, and my son, bless him, on becoming head boy at his junior school, was universally known as 'Head Chicken'.

I even called him that myself.

But if you are deranged enough to become a doctor . . .

I suppose it was preordained, really. I was born sometime before the Richard Gordon books, and my parents had resolved to call me Simon (I believe they were under some stress at the time) until a friend of my father's was killed in a motorcycle accident shortly before my christening. Bad news for him and his family, of course, but a blessing in disguise for me as Simon departed for ever, and Michael it was, in his memory.

My first acquaintance with the world of medicine took place when aged seven at my junior school. The teacher, a lean, earnest, bespectacled chap with thinning hair who seemed to me to be at least 140 but was probably in his early thirties, had an epileptic fit during a lesson and collapsed, frothing at the mouth, in front of the class.

Nobody moved for a while, least of all him, and then apparently I took myself off to the headmaster's study, strolled in unconcernedly and announced, 'Mr Seaman's dead, sir. Could we have someone else to finish the lesson?'

My father taught at the grammar school to which I ultimately went, which was interesting for us both, but probably the more painful for him, if I am honest.

5

I remember him describing to me an end-of-term staff meeting to choose the prefects for the forthcoming year. The headmaster, a grey-haired disciplinarian of the old school, announced firmly when my name came up for discussion, 'That boy will never become a prefect as long as I am in charge here.' My father was mortified, but I remember feeling strangely proud of this vote of no confidence in my abilities.

He was a gentle, scholarly man with a dry sense of humour. I can never once recall him raising his voice when dealing with a recalcitrant pupil – he had an altogether more subtle ploy up his sleeve.

All of us, even myself, had a healthy respect for the wrath of our headmaster. This was in the days when schoolmasters were still allowed to use the cane, and boy, was it a potent deterrent. The ultimate penalty for persistent offenders was to be sent to wait outside the headmaster's study during the course of a lesson. He had the eyes and ears of a hawk, and looked a bit like one too, with a long beaky nose and protruding eyes. He was possibly the forerunner of today's video security systems, because should you tiptoe up to the thick, heavy oak door of his study in stockinged feet and stand motionless outside, without breathing for minutes on end, he would always be unerringly aware of your presence. I think he must have smelled the sweat, and the fear.

The door would swing silently open, and he would beckon you ominously inside. A boy in the corridor during lesson time meant only one thing – or rather six of them – and discovery there led inevitably to a great deal of discomfort in the sitting department for the next few days.

Of course, the headmaster had other duties which led to him regularly being away from his office, and my father kept a meticulous diary of his daily activities. As I learned only after leaving school, he would never send a deserving case for his potential six of the best unless he knew full well that the headmaster was engaged elsewhere.

'Go and wait outside the head's study,' he would say sternly to the woeful miscreant, 'and come back here immediately the bell rings – not a minute before, you understand?'

The sheer terror instilled into an errant child, waiting timorously outside the door for a few swift but intensely painful moments of retribution, was infinitely worse than the swish of the cane itself.

'Never had to send the same boy twice,' admitted my father, smiling mischievously as he recounted this to me with relish.

I am not sure what it was that attracted me to medicine in those early days. It was certainly not the support and encouragement of colleagues of my father's, most of whom had known me since birth.

'Don't see why he couldn't do languages like his father,' I remember one of them grumbling, and he may have had a point save for the minor detail that I was inherently useless at them. The smell of formalin, I think, may have a lot to answer for, but then it may have been the time I came home at nine o'clock one evening, aged eleven, from playing football at our local youth club.

As I turned the corner into our road I saw my father being loaded into an ambulance and driven away, my mother and sister in tears on the doorstep. Nothing was said that night – I tried to stay awake until my mother returned from the hospital in the early hours, but fell asleep at about three in the morning.

The next day my mother would say little except that he was still alive, and to try not to worry too much, and it wasn't until halfway through the morning that another pupil enlightened me with the cheery words, 'Hear your dad's had a heart attack. He gonna snuff it, or what?'

Fortunately for now it was 'what', and not 'snuff it', but the spectre hung over us for years to come.

We all fondly remember our first love, as indeed do I – dissecting dogfish, earthworms and frogs in the biology lab – and it was this I suspect that drew me to a career in medicine. Not that there is an awful lot of call for carefully eviscerating an earthworm in general practice, these days.

We also kept and bred white rats, or did until we let all thirty of them out in the lab one day to allow them to explore new horizons only for the cleaner to open the lab door at an inopportune moment, thus allowing them all out to explore rather newer horizons than we had intended. I just hope it hurt the headmaster more when one of them bit him than it did us when he exacted his revenge sometime later.

There was no great medical precedent in our family for me to follow. My elder sister, Lesley, was the first to be led astray in the profession when she became a nurse, but by that stage it was too late to put me off. I duly set out on the round of medical school interviews, along with all the other poor deluded souls who felt that medicine offered them a life of professional satisfaction and personal fulfilment. Oh how young and innocent we all were . . .

I remember my first interview well. The brother of a boy in my year at school was 'studying' – I use the term loosely – at St Mary's Hospital Medical School, in Paddington. He was having such a whale of a time, apparently totally uninterrupted by work in any shape or form, that I resolved to go there immediately, without ever reading a single prospectus.

In any event I wanted to go to London, although the school and my father would have liked me to go to Cambridge, but it was an uneven contest between kudos for them, and sheer, undiluted entertainment for myself.

On university application forms in those days you had to stipulate five medical schools in order of preference. I put Mary's at number one, and bracketed four more random choices in the capital at number two. My intentions were set in stone – I was going to go to Mary's, whether they wanted me or not.

Most cities will only have one medical school to contend with, but London was blessed – or possibly cursed, dependent upon your point of view – with quite a few, each having its own distinctive characteristics.

You went to Guy's if you had a public school education, which luckily I didn't, St Thomas's if you thought you should have had a public school education but didn't, St Bartholomew's if your educational upbringing was immaterial because you were just naturally superior to all other life forms anyway, and George's if you were simply unable to get in anywhere else.

You opted for The Royal Free if you were a woman, or hoped that one day you might become one, and lastly St Mary's if you had no academic aspirations whatsoever but knew how to kick a rugby ball – yes, the women as well. You also went to Mary's if you were Welsh, being congenitally unable to master the underground system but possessing just enough intellectual capacity to stagger the two hundred yards from the mainline station to the medical school.

My first interview was at Mary's, lasted all of four minutes, and consisted of just three questions:

1. 'Did you have a good journey down?' Answer, 'Yes, thank you.'
2. 'What was the last book you read?' 'Winnie the Pooh.' (Well, it was!)
3. 'I see you played rugby for your county. Would you want to play for Mary's if you came here?' to which of course the answer was, 'Yes, I would love to.'

This was then followed by a spate of serious nodding all round. 'We'll see you next autumn, then,' they said, and I left with my place well and truly booked for the future.

Five years later, and it is finals time. With two of the four exams under my belt I develop a headache – not altogether an unusual experience in the life of a student, only this time alcohol plays no part in its acquisition. Worryingly, as I take my seat for the surgical paper, the headache is getting worse and worse, and I rest my head briefly on the desk, falling fast asleep. When I awake, I am in hospital with viral meningitis, all thoughts of qualification having disappeared into oblivion.

Two weeks pass, and whilst my friends are all out celebrating their newly found professional status I am at home, recovering, disillusioned, depressed, and still unable to drink enough alcohol to drown any of my considerable sorrows. For three months I refuse to open a textbook, and consider giving up my chosen career, and then, just as I am beginning to regain some sense of reason, tragedy strikes as my father drops dead from his final heart attack on the eighteenth hole of the golf course, in the late evening sun. What a way to go, but what sadness as he never lived long enough to see me qualify, one of his life's ambitions.

On the afternoon of his funeral I played golf on the same course, with a lump in my throat. All was well until I came to the eighteenth hole, an uphill par 4, and wouldn't you just know it but my second shot landed just inches from where he died. I walked up to where it lay, the tears flowing unashamedly down my cheeks, and stood there for a while, feeling closer to him in those few moments than I had in all the five years I had been away.

The next six months crawled by, my inclination to work having long disappeared, but I looked on the bright side. All my friends were wandering in complete exhaustion through hospital corridors in the early hours of the morning, and my golfing handicap had never been so good.

Resits finally arrived the following summer. I only had two exams left to pass – which was just as well, as to describe my medical knowledge at the time as being threadbare would be the understatement of the century. But the examiners were kind (or so I thought), and at last I emerged blinking into the sunlight with some real letters after my name.

My parents, obviously forward thinking, had added an 'Anthony' after the 'Michael' in my name so I could write my name as Sparrow, M. A. – 'Just in case you never manage to get a degree of your own,' said my father drily, but now I was Sparrow, MA, MBBS, LRCP, and no, I'm still not entirely sure what all the letters stand for, either.

I had passed, I always believed, due to having somehow acquired sufficient knowledge to scrape through the remaining two papers, but this happy state of self-delusion was brought abruptly to a halt by the Dean's secretary when I wandered into her office some years later on another matter entirely.

'We used to keep a black book on all our students,' she said, remembering fondly, 'listing their indiscretions whilst they were here. Some had hardly any entries, but yours . . . Would you like to see?' She grinned wickedly as I nodded out of sheer curiosity. 'Would you like to start with volume one, or volume two?'

I had qualified, I learned, thanks to the Professor of Surgery, a man whose fearsome reputation was equalled only by the glare on his face when a hapless student transgressed anywhere within his earshot.

'Get that man out of my hospital,' he had said at the post-exam meeting to discuss the fate of the borderline students. 'Pass him, if necessary.'

After qualification came the lull before the storm, a short holiday and a break from the mind-numbing boredom of revising subjects consisting of long words I was frequently unable even to pronounce correctly, let alone understand. And then you were pitched unawares into a maelstrom of activity the like of which you had never before encountered, where sleep became but a memory and life as you had known it was to vanish for eternity.

They call it 'house jobs.'

A house job is a six-month attachment as the most junior doctor in the hospital, a terrifying prospect at the best of times, and it derives its name from the fact that all the best students aim to work in the hospital in which they qualified. Certain jobs had huge prestige attached to them – working for the aforementioned Professor of Surgery, for example – and were vital for your future career. By agreeing to employ you, the medical school showed that it had a smattering of respect for your knowledge and abilities, and that no matter how abject you may have been at your chosen career you were in no respect as appalling as those dreadful individuals who ended up in peripheral hospitals well outside the capital.

Needless to say, I started my first job in the depths of south-east Kent, having not even bothered to apply for a post in the beloved institution of my training. My second house job was in a hospital in the north-west of England, where I arrived by one of those strange quirks of fate which so often shape our burgeoning medical development.

In the twilight world of the junior medic, trying to embark upon his as yet stuttering future career, the next job becomes an all-encompassing obsession. You arrive on the ward for the first time, introduce yourself to all the staff and then head off for the nearest phone to see who you can blackmail into employing you next, six months or even a year down the line.

I was, for once, rather lucky. My second post had been agreed on a handshake, and I had no such worries. At the end of my first six months' torture I got married, went on honeymoon, and came back, refreshed and ready for work. Life seemed at last to be easy, my career progressing according to plan – not a particularly good plan, it must be admitted, but at least a plan of my own making. I rang the consultant to see which day I should start.

His secretary was evasive. 'I'm not entirely sure where he is,' she would say each time I called.

'But you will see him,' I persisted. 'Please tell him I called and ask him to ring me back. I have to know when I am due to start.'

'I'll get him to call,' she promised.

After the eighth or ninth phone call the promises began to sound a little hollow. I resolved to take decisive action for a change, and drove to the hospital, some six hours distant from where I was staying with my newly acquired in-laws. After half an hour searching the corridors I finally tracked down the consultant

12

just as he was about to embark upon a ward round, complete with his fawning entourage.

It gives me scant satisfaction to recall that he shifted uneasily from foot to foot on my approach, looking nervously over his shoulder for some, indeed any, route of escape.

'My job,' I said firmly. 'You won't answer my calls, and I need to know – when would you like me to start?'

When you are young, and fresh-faced and innocent – as I think even I can lay claim to having been, at that time – consultants seem, and in reality frequently are, godlike creatures who can control your future, your success or your failure resting uneasily in the palms of their hands. He looked at me coldly over the rims of his half-moon glasses.

'Job?' he said, with studied indifference. 'And what job is that? There is no job for you here. I was unable to contact you, so I gave it to this young lady here, who at least I could rely upon to turn up when requested,' and he motioned towards a ravishingly beautiful young Eurasian girl standing dutifully by his side.

'But it was *my* job,' I said desperately, 'You promised it to *me*. I was on honeymoon, for God's sake. What on earth am I supposed to do now?'

Verging on the pathetic, I grant you, but that is precisely how I felt at that moment. Just married. No job, no home, and no money. No future.

He dismissed me with a casual wave of his hand. 'That is really not a problem I can trouble myself with, Dr Sparrow. You do not have a contract that I am aware of, whereas Dr Mather here . . .' resting a hand paternally on the young beauty's shoulder, who at least had the grace to look slightly discomforted, 'has one written in comparative tablets of stone. Now run away and bother somebody else with your troubles, there's a good boy. All of us here have some work to be getting along with, if you don't mind.'

For a few seconds a conviction for grievous bodily harm hung in the balance, but then I controlled myself, and left. It was a long time before I could view a senior surgeon again with anything but distaste.

There then followed ten days while I sat at my in-laws' house, fretting and waiting for the phone to ring, and just when I had all but given up hope my mother-in-law woke me early one morning with a smile on her face. I don't think I have ever seen it there since, but it was definitely there that day.

'It's the medical school for you,' she said. 'They've found you a job.'

A young doctor, just a week into his first post, had been tragically killed in a motorbike accident and they needed a replacement, and for the second time in my life somebody else's misfortune had been to my advantage.

House jobs could be, and frequently were, the nearest thing to hell on earth most of us will encounter. The sleep deprivation can border on the suicidal – I once worked from a Thursday morning to a Monday evening without ever going to bed, or as far as I know even to sleep. It was the stuff of nightmares, and not only for ourselves.

The patients surely had some right to expect the doctor attending them to be capable of the odd rational thought process, and committed to attending to their medical and personal needs. What we really wanted, of course, was to bundle them out of the bed they had just arrived in so we could crawl in ourselves, and get some rest.

But somehow you survive it, using up several lifetimes' supply of adrenaline and acquiring the art of cat-napping between sentences. It is thankfully no longer so bad these days, but on the plus side it taught us how to cope with almost anything that would later be thrown at us. For me, it seemed that there was an awful lot out there just waiting to be launched in my direction.

Throughout my second house job my thoughts were constantly turning to my future. Never again did I want to be put in the position of having no job to go to when the current one expired, and so, for some reason I still cannot understand, I joined the air force.

I can, I should explain, fully understand why I applied – a guaranteed job for the next five years, and I like to think I've always looked good in blue. I just can't understand why they accepted me.

The interview was interesting. I had very long hair, a very short attention span, and a very limited idea of what the air force was all about. The whole affair took about an hour, but I can only recall one question. Around the walls of the interview room were various pictures of fast jets, a couple of which I later came to actually fly. One of the panel, a real gentleman of a Group Captain who was obviously interested in the depth of my knowledge regarding my forthcoming employers, asked me if I could identify any of them.

I considered long and hard. Some sort of intelligent response was clearly required.

'Well,' I said eventually, 'that one's a blue one, that is a white one, and that one over there has a lot of camouflagey bits on it.'

Looking back after all these years, I can think of only one reason why they accepted me.

They were desperate.

I spent, eventually, six years in the RAF, and finally left by mutual agreement. I wanted to go, and they were equally keen to get rid of me.

My wife was born and bred in West Devon, and had always wanted to return home – sometimes, I like to think, even wanting me to go with her. We had spent most of our brief holidays in the area, and to be honest I loved the place, so making the decision to move there was the easy bit. Finding a job was rather more difficult.

General practice posts in Devon were highly sought after, and good references (something the RAF had neglected to provide for me) an essential element to procuring the job of your dreams.

Sure, I had local knowledge, and contacts, but vacancies were scarce. What was needed was just that little bit of luck.

It came, as so often, in the early hours of the morning, and in a pub. My late father-in-law, Charles, a wonderful character with a reputation that spread across several counties, had a comprehensive knowledge of the public houses of Devon, and an instinct of long standing for which of them would be still open after hours.

A generous-spirited man, he had a host of friends and acquaintances who also liked to spend the early hours of the morning propping up a bar, and one such night found us in the Buller's Arms, a picturesque establishment in one of the local villages.

'So you want to come down here to work, then?' said a grey-haired lady in her early sixties, tossing down a gin and tonic with considerable relish. 'Best try Dr Margaret, if you ask me. Rushed off her feet, she is, most of the time. If ever a woman needed a partner, she does, even if it is . . .' eyeing me up doubtfully, 'someone who looks as disreputable as you.'

So saying, she threw her head back and roared with laughter, whilst I laughed too. It seemed like the polite thing to do.

Dr Margaret was the remaining half of Dr Christopher and Dr Margaret, Dr Christopher having expired during morning surgery some five years earlier. It says much about Margaret's character that she took a deep breath, shed a tear or two, and then went off and finished surgery for him.

'Well, he wouldn't have wanted it any other way,' she told me once, many years later. 'And in any case, they would only have come back in the evening . . .'

Margaret and Christopher had arrived in the village of Lifton in 1954, and stayed ever since. They had become an institution. Gradually, as other doctors in the area had reached retirement, they had taken over their practices as well and dedicated their whole lives to meeting the needs of the local population.

After Christopher's death, Margaret had worked alone, but the pressures of the changing health service, and her increasing age (although nobody, not even her daughter, was exactly sure how old she was) were beginning to take their toll. Everyone I spoke to confirmed that first opinion – Margaret needed a partner, and needed one soon.

This should be pretty easy, I thought, so I wrote to her, offering my services.

She turned me down flat.

I wrote to her again, and she turned me down even more flatly, and so I wrote to her once more, saying that if she ever needed a locum, I would be happy to help out in any way I could. I even volunteered to cut her grass and do the shopping, which can only be described as abject grovelling. When she wrote back, I could see she was already beginning to weaken.

Margaret was a small, fiercely determined lady with a tremendous sense of discipline (oh, we were so well suited) who looked just like the Queen. She interviewed me one day after morning surgery, and I must have really wanted the job because I had my hair cut, wore a suit, and didn't smoke or swear once during the entire proceedings. In fact, I was in such awe of her that it was more than three years before she saw me with a cigarette in my hand at all.

On that occasion we were both out walking our dogs down the lane from the surgery, she on the way out, and I on the way back. Lost in a world of my own, I was within a yard of her before I sensed her presence at all. Hastily, I held the cigarette behind my back, pathetically trying to hide its existence.

We stood in the evening sunshine and chatted for a few moments, the cigarette burning lower and lower down towards the butt, and then smoke started creeping up my back and drifting in little wisps over my shoulder. Margaret appeared not to notice, and I breathed a sigh of relief and moved on.

A few yards further down the lane I heard her voice floating behind me: 'I should put that cigarette out before it burns a hole in your hand, if I were you.'

The interview was more of a gentle chat between colleagues than anything, a very low-key affair. Afterwards I emerged blinking into the sunshine, somewhat bemused by the speed of the turn of events. One minute I was an all but unemployed ex-air force doctor with a questionable set of references and the next I had landed a plum position in a highly sought-after part of the country. I was now in possession of something I had vaguely heard of but thought only others were ever likely to acquire: prospects.

I can no longer remember what I did with them, but I do know they were there for a while. What I did not have, however, was a house, or any money, or any idea as to how I was going to lay my hands upon either.

Margaret, bless her, was an extremely well-off country GP approaching the end of her career who had a totally unrealistic concept of what an impecunious young doctor such as myself could afford. She suggested I take a look at some of the finer local residences, which I did, but after due reflection I merely considered applying for the post of the second under-gardener, calculating accurately that he would probably be on a higher wage scale than myself for the next few years. I asked her how much she thought it might cost, and tried not to gulp too much when she told me.

I then asked her if she knew of any nearby sheds with corrugated roofs that didn't leak too much, or if she wasn't using her garage every night of the week could I have it on the particularly rainy days.

I think she thought that I was joking.

As I stood in her drive, wondering if my mother had ever disposed of the tent we had had when my sister and I were younger, I noticed that across the road a solitary red-haired figure was standing on a newly cleared piece of land, holding a brick.

18

With that flash of inspiration that years of rigorous training had so firmly instilled into me, I surmised that he might be a builder, that the brick might one day become a house, and that the house might be in need of an occupant. I wandered casually across the road.

'Morning,' I said politely. 'Building here?'

The red-headed man looked from brick to me and after due consideration finally pronounced, 'Yup.'

'A house?' I inquired tentatively, half expecting some such facetious answer as 'No, a shopping complex, actually.'

'Yup,' he responded again.

'Got a buyer?' I continued casually.

There was a short pause whilst his brow furrowed, a change of reply being needed here. 'Nope,' he said eventually, having considered all the relevant options.

'And how much will it be, then, when it's finished?'

He scratched his head thoughtfully, looked me up and down rather more shrewdly than I would have previously given him credit for, and named a figure.

'Fine,' I said, more nonchalantly than I felt. 'I'll take it, then.'

He held out his hand and inspected his palm, and for one awful moment I thought he was going to spit on it and I would have to try my luck elsewhere. Thankfully, however, he just rubbed it briskly on his trousers a couple of times (they were a good deal more dirty than his hand was, but it's the thought that counts) and we shook on the deal.

No contracts, no arguments on either side, no later haggling over any details, and no delays of any sort. The whole process had taken less than three minutes.

They do things differently, in the country.

So there I was, in Lifton, and here I have remained for the past twelve years.

It is a small village of around a thousand inhabitants, situated just east of the Devon–Cornwall border. When I arrived, the main road into Cornwall ran right through the village centre, splitting it in two – but it's OK, you can breathe easily now. They have since built a bypass, and you can drive right past us without ever knowing we were there.

It took a while to settle into country life, and get used to the characters who lived there. To one who was a 'townie' at heart, farmers had always been those people who reported you to your parents for playing in their barns without permission, but now they formed a large part of my practice.

There was one in particular, Tom, a good friend of Charles (my father-in-law), who did a splendid interpretation of all the calls of a hunting horn and delighted in buying you whisky after whisky, shoving you from one end of the bar to the other whilst he was doing so. They staggered home together one evening after a lengthy session in one of the local hostelries, and Charles bade Tom farewell at the gate, turning to walk away.

Unfortunately, it was the wrong gate, and Tom duly turned around, took a couple of slightly unsteady steps forward, and fell head first into the silage pit in the field immediately opposite his house. They must share the blame between them for my complete inability to look a glass of whisky in the face for the past fifteen years.

And then there was Martin, a droll, ruddy-faced farmer with an impenetrable Devon accent who once bet the entire pub that he could get a snooker ball in his mouth and close his lips fully around it. Which he could . . . but sadly was unable to open his jaws wide enough to get it out again.

The surgery was in fact part of Margaret's house, and was tiny, with barely enough room for us both to work in at the same time. I knew that one day she would have to retire, and equally knew that she would put off the dreaded day until the last possible moment. I reckoned that I would have probably six or seven years to decide where I was going to practise from when her house became no longer available.

The bombshell arrived six months after starting to work.

The government of the day brought in a compulsory retirement age of seventy for all GPs, and Margaret was already beyond the limit – although by just how far, nobody was able to tell. Together we managed to persuade the health authority to grant her a one-year stay of execution because of our particular circumstances, but I had been suddenly presented with a nightmare scenario.

Everything in the surgery belonged to Margaret – I had no drugs, no equipment, and no money to acquire either, and worst of all was soon to be faced with the small matter of no surgery to work from. Building sites in Lifton were scarce, as the property boom at the time had meant every square inch of the village that was suitable had already been developed.

Every square inch but one.

I bought – with the not inconsiderable help of an amazingly understanding bank manager – the old piggery next to Margaret's house, which, as luck would have it, was owned by Margaret in the first place. The next year was spent frantically building, and finally the new surgery was ready, and only three months after it was meant to be, too.

It was at least four or five times as big as its predecessor. I can remember wandering around it on my own, the evening before opening for business, wondering what on earth I was going to do with all the rooms I had to play with. Twelve years later we now wander around aimlessly, wondering where on earth we are going to put everything.

Gradually, I began to modernise the practice. I was forty years younger than Margaret, and had my own ideas as to how the surgery should be run, only now there had been a subtle but significant change in our relationship. Margaret – although helping me out part-time, without which I would never have coped at all – was still smarting from having to retire. I had become the 'boss', such as it was, instead of the very much junior partner, and we both struggled at first to come to terms with the shifting emphasis.

In those days there were no co-operatives of GPs helping each other cover the out-of-hours work – nights and weekends – and there was a scarcity of locums available, particularly in the West Country. As Margaret's health began to fail, it was obvious that I needed some assistance on a full-time basis.

Old receptionists were replaced by new, and I introduced computers for the first time. None of us had the least idea how to use them, but they looked impressive, sitting there in the corner and gathering dust.

Next, I brought in a practice nurse. Margaret had always dealt with all the standard nursing procedures, but I was congenitally incapable of applying even a piece of sticking plaster to the tiniest of wounds, let alone knowing what to do with a bandage, a poultice, or any of the other messy bits and pieces that nurses are so good at. Ideally I tried not to touch the patient at all, especially if they smelt a bit funny, and so into the practice came Catherine, dark-haired, stubborn, feisty and of Irish extraction, who has been invaluable ever since. We might argue vociferously on occasion, but I always manage to see her point of view in the end, before ignoring it completely.

Two years later Margaret was now terminally ill, and unable to help any longer. She died in the end whilst I was on holiday in Kenya, being buried the day before my return.

The practice had grown steadily throughout this time, and there was now more work than I could readily handle. I was exhausted, and in any case needed someone else with whom to share the blame when everything went pear-shaped.

Word went out that I was looking for a partner.

There were a surprising number of very kind GPs who decided to come calling, offering to take the reins from the hands of a poor innocent GP they thought obviously incapable of surviving on his own. They were however firmly rebuffed until I met Dr Harper, who seemed perfect.

For a start, he looked even less like a doctor than I did. An eccentric mad professor, certainly, with bits of hair sticking out all over the place, and arms and legs that apparently moved independently both of each other and of any rational thought processes. More importantly, he not only knew how to turn the computer on, but how to put snippets of information on it. What more could I ask?

Talking to Dr Harper was, and remains, an interesting experience. You can go to ask him a question, and spend twenty minutes discussing something totally unrelated before departing not only without getting an answer, but having completely forgotten what it was you went to ask him in the first place. It is perfect for general practice in the country – the patients come in, spend half an hour in his consulting room, and then depart with absolutely no idea what it was they were ill with when they arrived there.

So that is Lifton, a small rural backwater that has remained unchanged for the twelve years of my working there, a tranquil idyll in a busy world, where nothing out of the ordinary ever seems to happen, and life in general practice continues uninterrupted by incident of any sort.

But back to the beginning . . .

2

Early Days at Medical School

Arriving at medical school was an eye-opening experience.

I had taken a year off following A-levels, resolving to travel the world and 'find' myself. But my father's health had taken a turn for the worse and I decided to stay at home instead.

A pity, really, because he recovered and sailed through the year in splendid fashion, and I have never managed to find myself since.

I could have skied in the Alps, mountain trekked in the Himalayas, swum in shark-infested waters in Central America . . . instead I found myself working for a firm of accountants in Wellingborough, Northants, the only occupation I know that makes biochemistry look interesting. It was however an invaluable grounding for later life, as general practice has become ever more of a business to be run like any other.

But at last it was day one at St Mary's. All the new intake of students were congregated in the canteen, a large room in the bowels of the building that was to become our second home. Here we would meet each morning (sometimes through the simple expedient of having failed to get out of there the night before) and seek sanctuary between those lectures we bothered to turn up to.

Everyone was nervously talking to everyone else, and occasionally listening. I looked around curiously. These people were going to be my colleagues, and some of them my friends, for the next five years of my life. God, what a prospect.

'Of course, I've always wanted to be a cardio-thoracic surgeon,' said an earnest, bespectacled lad in a light grey jacket to my left, looking as if he needed to reach puberty first. 'And today I really feel I'm beginning to live that dream.'

'Well, that's him off my list of interesting people to get stuck in a lift with, for a start,' murmured a voice in my ear, and I turned to see a Jools Holland look-alike smiling mischievously by my side. This was Neil – 'Shortknees', as he was universally to be known due to his diminutive stature, and destined to be a flatmate of the future. Not so much a case of love at first sight, but more to do with the fact that we awoke side by side, following a little gentle over-indulgence on Freshers' Night, wondering what we were doing asleep under the sinks in the ladies' loo.

Gradually, over the next few weeks, the sea of faces began to develop names and characters, and cliques of like-minded people began to drift together – the rugby players, the boffins, anyone with glasses, those with a criminal record . . .

I lived at first in a large, single-sex hall of residence near King's Cross, which had three other students from Mary's. There was Ken, an amiable, cherubic-faced Midlander; Tony, known universally as TCA – his initials standing for tricarboxylic acid, a compound we were to become unbearably acquainted with in subsequent biochemistry lessons – who wandered around with a constant look of bemusement on his face; and Dave, a red-headed Northerner.

Then there was Roger, who lived in the mixed hall of residence next door (lucky boy). Tall, blond, blue-eyed and handsome, he subsidised his way through medical school by becoming a sperm donor – occasionally even to the fertility clinics.

Another hall of residence a quarter of a mile down the road housed a fellow soccer player, Polson, the aforementioned Shortknees, and 'Skid' Kellegher, so named because of his ill-fated attempt to drive home after the Freshers' Night party in our first week.

Freshers' Night, I should explain, is a ritual introduction to the newly arrived students that requires all concerned to drink to great excess and forget all the inhibitions they ever had. And given the broad spectrum of those inhibitions in the first place, you can begin to get the idea as to the quantities of alcohol this might entail.

Whilst the rest of us staggered off in what we vaguely hoped might be our homeward direction, Skid decided to drive, despite our repeated protestations and dire warnings of what damage he might wreak upon himself, let alone the other hapless inhabitants of London. But we need not have worried, because he never made it out of the car park, wrapping his car round a bollard just a matter of yards from where he was parked. He never even had chance to get out of second gear, and just sat there for a while, spinning his wheels furiously in an effort to escape.

The five-year stint at medical school is split into two unequal halves, pre-clinical – a two- year sentence – and clinical, which is three. In our pre-clinical stage we are safely kept away from all patients, or at least those that are still alive, and study anatomy, physiology, biochemistry and pharmacology, with an exam in each subject at the end of each year.

The first-year exam is known as 1st MB, and the second, strangely enough, as 2nd MB, and yes, it is almost as boring to do as it is for you to read about.

In our clinical years, should we survive that far – and by no means everyone does – we get to touch the public, although mostly in places we would each rather we didn't have to. Here we study medicine, surgery, obstetrics and gynaecology, therapeutics and pathology, the last of these almost as mind-numbingly boring as biochemistry – so boring, in fact, that Shortknees, myself and a couple of friends decided to go to France for a few weeks instead, and nobody noticed. Exams come at monotonously regular intervals, with finals, the ultimate hurdle of them all, lying ominously in wait for us, five years down the road.

There is a touching faith in the non-medical fraternity that students mysteriously transform into doctors due to their extensive knowledge of medicine, their razor-sharp clinical acumen and their deep insight into the human psyche.

But I have to disillusion you. It's just not true.

Times have changed since the freewheeling, carefree days of medical students in the late seventies and early eighties. For a start, students actually have to learn something, these days. They also have to suffer the Chinese water torture of continual assessment instead of months, or even years, of masterly inactivity culminating in sustained and frantic last-minute cramming for exams.

Transmitting your knowledge to the examiners – or attempting to disguise your lack of it – can be a nerve-racking business. This is particularly true in vivas – the Latin name for the oral exams – where two sadistic torturers endeavour to ask you questions about branches of medicine you have never even heard of.

Sometimes, however, it doesn't quite get that far.

A friend of mine, a highly talented rugby player but an amiably lackadaisical student with only a passing acquaintance of the subject in hand, was approaching his final viva at the end of the second-year exams. He knew that he had done a less than impressive written paper, and that realistically his chances of passing the viva, and with it progression to the heady heights of the clinical years, were limited.

As he walked across the examination room to meet his fate, his heart sank. There were always two examiners for these joyous occasions – one internal, from your own medical school, and one external examiner from a completely inferior medical school somewhere else in the country whose prime responsibility – supposedly – was to ensure that candidates were neither unfairly discriminated against nor promoted beyond their abilities.

The internal examiner was the Professor of Embryology, renowned for his feverish enthusiasm for all things embryological and his equally feverish distaste for all things rugby-playing. He could not understand why grown men should wish to run around in the autumnal mud throwing oval balls at each other when they could be furthering their knowledge in his own particular speciality. Unsurprisingly he was always fiercely antagonistic to such participants during their exams.

The professor – a small, bespectacled, energetic little man – was seated behind a trestle table upon which lay his prized embryological exhibits, all neatly displayed to show off their most favourable aspects. They were generally unidentifiable bits of tissue suspended in blocks of plastic with unintelligible names and supremely complicated origins. He cherished them like children.

'Irreplaceable, my dear boy,' he would chatter as he cooed paternally over them. 'Quite irreplaceable – don't come too close, now. Don't want you running the risk of breaking them, ha ha.'

The professor's second love, however, was sherry, and he was well known for his habit of imbibing one or two glasses during the lunchtime recess. It was Friday, the last day of the exams, there were only a few poor students left to interrogate, and he had imbibed aplenty. Colin was the first victim after his quietly over-indulgent lunch, and as he and the professor were not on the best of terms, his prospects seemed grim.

But here fate lent a hand. As Colin neared the table the professor rose to greet him with a steely glint in his eye.

A rugby player, he was probably thinking, and one I dislike intensely, to boot. This should be fun.

His knee caught the corner of the table as he got to his feet, the exhibits shook and rattled ominously, and in what Colin described as the slowest of slow motion the most prized of all his specimens toppled towards the floor. Colin – not even by his closest friends' assessment the most academically alert individual – was nonetheless physically gifted beyond the average.

He dived forward and threw himself full length along the ground, clutching the priceless antiquity in his outstretched hands just inches before it would have smashed irrevocably on the dissection room floor.

The professor sprang round the table, dancing a little jig of undiluted joy. 'Splendid, oh splendid, my boy,' he chortled. 'Oh very good indeed. My prize exhibit. Irreplaceable, utterly irreplaceable. Quite splendid of you.'

He subsided in due course, and looked at his saviour benignly. 'Well, Mr Walsh,' he chirruped, 'do let us begin. I have a feeling you are going to do well, very well indeed.'

Needless to say, Colin passed, and with flying colours.

'The easiest viva imaginable,' was his bemused comment as he emerged with a look of wonder on his face. 'I just wonder what would have happened if I had dropped it.'

But it was not always that way. There was the case of John, a student in my year with a very distinctive surname, who was quiet, unassuming, well mannered, diligent and knowledgeable. What he was doing at St Mary's Hospital, Paddington, remains one of the unexplained mysteries of life.

He was supremely uninterested in rugby, or drinking regularly to excess, or indeed pursuing anything in a skirt, a starched uniform or with child-bearing potential – an apparent prerequisite for all Mary's students – and was confidently and justifiably expected by all to sail through his 2nd MB with the minimum of difficulty.

Until, that is, he met his Nemesis – in the shape of the external examiner in the anatomy viva.

John walked in his usual unassuming manner down to where the examiners were waiting, and took his seat. The external examiner was perusing his list of candidates.

'Ah,' he said, with a slight curl of his lip, 'you are Mr—, are you? An unusual name – tell me,' and he took off his glasses and laid them slowly and deliberately on the table, 'are you by any chance related to a certain—?'

John took a deep breath. 'He was my father,' he said simply.

His father, I should say, had been involved in a major political scandal some years previously, which even now occasionally hits the newspaper headlines.

The examiner smiled, baring his teeth in wolverine fashion. 'I lost a lot of money, thanks to your father,' he said, raising his papers. 'Now, let us see what sort of material the son is made of . . .'

The student, need I add, subsequently failed. The only comment I ever heard him make was a philosophical, 'But I'm used to it.'

The examiner, no doubt, felt that a belated piece of justice had been done. Such is the power of one in his position.

There was another examiner on the circuit with his own particular brand of humour, and I might have thought this an apocryphal tale had I not heard it from several unimpeachably different sources.

Examinations always took place in the summer, and for some inexplicable reason the day of the vivas would always herald clear blue skies and uninterrupted sunshine, as if Mother Nature herself was mocking those for whom the Sword of Damocles was personally hovering.

For some poor candidates, this particular examiner would rise at the end of the viva and lead them across to the window, a fatherly arm around their shoulders.

'You see those trees,' he would say benignly. 'Look at the leaves, how very green they are, and how delightfully they catch the sun. You rejoice in the glories of Mother Nature like myself, do you not?'

The student would nod sympathetically in agreement, no doubt expecting some analogy to the blossoming beauty of their own career. The examiner would then turn to look at them, staring deeply into their eyes.

'Those leaves will be brown when you return for your resits,' he would say chillingly, 'and I will look forward to seeing you in the autumn . . .'

In complete contrast to this, my anatomy viva at the end of the first year was a rather enjoyable affair.

I knew I had passed the written paper – our Professor of Anatomy would give us oblique cryptic clues to the forthcoming questions, and having spent much of the first year in the students' canteen applying myself with vigour to all the crosswords I could lay my hands upon, I had guessed the paper accurately and learned the answers accordingly.

Unfortunately, I hadn't learned anything else, so for the viva I adopted a different approach. I took a deep breath and trusted to luck.

Due to the sudden illness of the external examiner I was blessed with the good fortune to have two members of the St Mary's medical staff asking me the questions. The Professor of Anatomy was one, but to my horror the other was the senior neurophysiologist whose dislike for me was equalled only by my distaste for him. It was he who was due to ask me the questions, and I resigned myself to fate, and the autumn leaves.

But then my guardian angel lent a hand.

The Professor of Anatomy, Mr Menzies, was a dour Scot with a wickedly dry sense of humour. For reasons nobody knew he always wore a white shirt and red tie, and he was the only man I ever met who could make an anatomy lecture both interesting and funny. Unusually, he and I got on extremely well. At the end of the second year, for example, I approached him one day with a list of the six questions which I thought might constitute the written exam.

'I do know I shouldn't be showing you this,' I said tentatively. 'But if this isn't the anatomy paper this year, then I am not going to be a student here next . . .'

He stood and looked at me for a moment, totally impassive. 'You're right,' he said at length, 'you shouldn't be showing me this. Do you understand what it would mean if I should pass any comment, and someone were to find out?'

I nodded, barely trusting myself to speak.

'Well, as long as that's understood then,' he said finally,

'the first five are right. Take another guess at question number six.'

As I took my seat in front of the pair of them, Menzies put his hand across the neuro-physiologist's chest, as if restraining him from crossing the road in front of oncoming traffic, and growled, 'I think I'll do this one, Dr Heath, if you don't mind.'

I rather think Dr Heath did mind. He looked as if he would have been only too pleased to have had the opportunity to establish the gaps in my knowledge, and would be sadly let down by having such an appetising prospect whisked away from him. He gave way with barely concealed disgust, however, and Mr Menzies began.

He leaned forward and rummaged among the haphazard pile of anatomical specimens before him, emerging with his prize like a keen bargain hunter at the local church jumble sale.

'Nae then, young Sparrow,' he said, 'can ye no tell me what this is?'

It was definitely a human bone, I knew that. And a big one. I considered carefully.

'No,' I replied truthfully.

Dr Heath raised his eyes to the ceiling.

'OK then,' conceded Mr Menzies, putting what was in fact the femur down and lifting up what even I could recognise as being a complete left foot, 'but you can tell me what this is, I trust?'

I nodded, relaxing a little. Safe ground here. 'A left foot, sir.'

'Very good, laddie,' he continued with heavy sarcasm. 'Nae, can ye tell me which bone in the foot this one is?' tapping it with a gnarled forefinger.

'No,' I replied.

'Or this?' he continued encouragingly, prodding another.

'Er . . . no,' I repeated in a small voice.

'Can ye no tell me the name of *any* bone in this foot, then?' he said, a touch exasperated.

Even I was beginning to feel sorry for myself. Feet were obviously not my strong point.

'No,' I whispered, hoping this torture would end as quickly as possible.

Dr Heath, who had been drumming the table in frustration, suddenly ceased abruptly and arose. 'I think I'll go for a walk,' he said tersely. 'I'm not sure I can take all this,' and he strode off round the examination room in search of more worthy opponents.

Mr Menzies looked at me again. 'Right, laddie,' he grunted, 'let's start afresh, shall we? And just you remember that I'm in charge here, will you? Nae then,' raising the aforementioned left foot once more and indicating another bone, 'see if you can tell me whether this is the talus.'

I regarded him cautiously. Was this a trick question?

'The answer begins with a "Y",' he continued with a sigh.

'Yes?' I ventured tentatively.

'Splendid, laddie. At last we seem to be getting somewhere. Now is this . . .' more prodding, '. . . the navicular?' and he shook his head slowly from side to side.

'No,' I answered more confidently.

'Very good. Ye're learning laddie, at last.' He put the foot down, its task completed, and continued, 'Now, tell me. Which of these bones here on the table is the radius?'

I was learning, all right. I waited for his lead, and sure enough he reached forward, grasped my hand and placed it firmly on one of the thin bones in front of us.

'This one,' I said, 'not a doubt about it . . .'

I passed.

Now this may, to you, seem rather a strange way to conduct the examinations of the young men and women who will one day carry the responsibility of being your surgeons, gynaecologists, GPs, etc, and in truth – of course it is. Many students in this early stage of their careers are, like myself, woefully lacking in knowledge relating to their chosen profession.

Others have facts coming out of their ears and overflowing into the ashtrays.

The unpalatable truth is that a good student does not necessarily make an excellent doctor, nor a bad student an awful one. Having survived the battlefield that constitutes the rat race of entry into medical school, we are all pretty much capable of acquiring the requisite knowledge and clinical expertise to become more than acceptable doctors . . .

We just do it at different stages of our careers, that's all.

Mr Menzies, I believe, looked for other qualities in his students than merely the ability to reproduce a stream of studiously learned facts like parrots in a memory competition. He sought for honesty, a sense of humour and perspective, an innate ability to survive the undoubted traumas and stresses of a life in medicine, and courage in the face of adversity.

At least, that's my excuse, and I'm sticking to it.

And then eventually came finals, and Mrs Axworthy.

I was not, we have established, the most knowledgeable of students. If ever a man was destined for the autumn leaves, then I was he. When resits came along, following my temporary leave of absence with meningitis, I had vague expectations in surgery, but none whatsoever in medicine. I think it fair to say that this was a completely justified assessment shared by both my colleagues and my tutors.

I had, by some fluke of nature, negotiated the written paper in medicine without total disaster. Any other student would have cautiously anticipated a pass, but I was more realistic. This was based upon the philosophical reflection that I didn't actually know anything, and had only a passing acquaintance with real patients.

For some unaccountable reason – an inherent obsession in the pursuit of lost causes, perhaps – I decided to turn up for the second part of the examination. This is the filling in the sandwich between written and oral tests, when we get to interrogate real patients with real diseases, and have some forty minutes to learn all there is to know of their lives, pathology, and TV viewing habits. We are left alone with the poor object of our attentions and at the end of the allotted time – oh, joy – the examiners return to quiz us on our newly acquired knowledge.

This is followed by four to six 'spot' cases, involving end of the bed diagnoses and a few subsequent questions. Do well in the long case and you should be laughing.

I arrived at the examination room and was shown through to where two stern-looking consultants stood waiting, resplendent in their spotless white coats. A little old lady was seated to one side.

'This is Mrs Axworthy,' announced one of my soon-to-be inquisitors, 'and she has an interesting tale to tell.' My reputation – or comparative lack of it – must have preceded me, because he added, 'We shall be intrigued to see how little of it you can present to us.'

They left. Mrs Axworthy looked at me sympathetically.

'You poor dear,' she said kindly. 'They don't seem to like you very much, do they? Seen it before, you know – bring me here every year, they do. Cup of tea and a biscuit and yer bus fare home and they think they own you. I'm one o' their regulars, don't you know.'

'You mean you only get your bus fare?' I asked, all thoughts of passing long dispensed with. No point in asking any medical questions, I realised. I just wouldn't know what to do with the answers. 'Don't you get a fee or anything? My God, are they exploiting you too?'

'Bless you, me dear,' she wheezed. 'It's a day out, and I get so few o' them, these days. Nice of you to think of it, though.'

She looked to the left, and to the right. Is this an important physical sign? I thought absently, having not a clue what it might signify, and then she beckoned me towards her with an arthritic finger.

I bent down to listen.

'Check the doors,' she whispered conspiratorially. 'Stick yer 'ead out. Go and make sure they've gone – they listen outside sometimes. Go on now, do as I tell you.'

I acquiesced, crept to the door obediently and cautiously looked out into the corridor. I hadn't a clue why I was doing it, but it was much more fun than talking medicine. I crept back.

'Coast is clear,' I ventured, wondering if she had a hip flask secreted about her person and needed some privacy to imbibe from it. 'What do we do now?'

She reached forward and grasped my collar. 'Listen to me,' she said, a misty look in her eyes. 'This'll be my last year, and you will be my last student. I'm too old now, and too ill. I won't make it here again, and I've had so many happy times with you young reprobates.'

She chuckled suddenly, a mischievous look flitting across her wrinkled face. 'Oh, I've had some fun with you students. Specially the pompous ones, misled 'em a treat, I have, when I've a mind to.'

Twenty minutes gone, I thought wryly. This was more fun than *Fawlty Towers*.

'But you're all right, dear,' she added, a tear in her eye. 'I like you. Bet you don't know nothing, but it don't matter ter me. Them professors an' all, they know everything there is about medicine, maybe. Can't talk to us patients, though, not proper like. You're all right, you are.'

She subsided into her memories for a moment as I stood there, wondering what was to come next, and then she shivered, as if recalling a whole load of pompous predecessors and the unpleasant taste they had left in her mouth. I waited patiently, knowing I had nothing to lose, and then she waved me towards a supermarket bag in the corner of the room.

'Bring us that, luv, there's a dear.'

I obeyed without question, and handed her the bag.

'Is it your tablets?' I asked 'Do you need one of those heart ones? Are you OK?'

She laughed throatily. 'Bless you, me ducks. You'll be the death of me. This is for you, me dear, with me blessing.'

She reached into the bag and pulled out a sheaf of papers. 'It's all here,' she continued, suddenly brisk and businesslike. 'All typed out by me niece. Me medical history, me diseases, all them drugs I'm on and their side effects. All them signs an' symptoms an' things you're s'posed to know.

'An' this,' she winked at me asthmatically, 'is a list of all them questions they ask, and all the right answers. So predictable, them consultants, an' they don't like you much, do they? I can tell, you know, but they forgets us exhibits. I've got me feelings, too. Now dear, twenty minutes, that's what you got to learn it all. Go on, get reading, it's all you'll need. I'll be 'aving a little nap, if yer don't mind.'

And she closed her eyes, a contented smile on her face, and slept peacefully while I read, scarcely believing my good fortune. I passed, thanks to Mrs Axworthy, and was glad that she had gone out in such a blaze of glory.

I owe her much.

There is a footnote to this tale which I learned some years later. The following year, now in desperate ill health, Mrs Axworthy apparently returned for a final triumphant performance. A friend of mine, who was even less academically gifted than myself, encountered her in his long case, much as I had. She dispatched him, too, to the corridor, and passed across her sheet of instructions, but such was his nervousness that he felt it necessary to nip to the loo and spent the next twenty-five minutes there, reading avidly. He arrived back just in advance of the return of the examiners to find Mrs Axworthy still and lifeless in her chair, mouth open and smiling serenely.

'And what can you tell us about this lovely lady?' oozed the Professor of Medicine dangerously, blissfully unaware of the tragic circumstances. My friend looked across at her, and then back to his inquisitor, and took a deep breath.

'She's dead, sir,' he said with great aplomb.

It was probably the most medically accurate statement he had made in his career to that date. It was indisputably true.

He passed. How could they possibly fail him?

I'm sure Mrs Axworthy would have approved.

3

The Art of Delivery

Babies.

We've all been one, but somehow this reassuring fact is of little practical help when we are faced with the labouring mother-to-be screaming, 'I can't stand it any more,' the concerned father dabbing ineffectually at any bit of his partner that comes within reach of his damp flannel, and the baby that just does not want to come out.

'Do something, doctor,' they all chorus, and you finally realise that what they were trying to teach you as a student – echoes of Tony Blair here – 'Deliver, deliver, deliver,' was actually quite sensible advice, not merely an attempt to reduce the joy in your life by insisting upon attendance in the ward when you would rather be somewhere, indeed anywhere, else.

My introduction to the obstetric unit demonstrated how easy it can be to lose your way in a strange environment. But it wasn't my fault. I had only been at Mary's for three and a half years – how could I possibly have been expected to know my way around the place by then?

In my third year at medical school I used to live in a flat in Kilburn. Interesting place, Kilburn, in those days. It had everything a man could desire. A Chinese takeaway, for a start – they might be everywhere nowadays but back in the seventies they were like gold dust, only more affordable. It also boasted an excellent bus service (something that lives on only in the memory after twelve years in the rural south west) and a whole host of pubs that no sane Englishman would ever dream of setting foot into.

Most sinister of these was Biddy Mulliner's, a devoutly Irish establishment that had once been bombed and was invariably full of black-bereted, pockmarked, silent individuals whose very presence just dared you to enter the portals.

We dared not.

We did however occasionally venture into one of the pubs further down the road, the only one I have ever frequented with real sawdust on the floors, and bloodstains on the walls . . .

Best of all we lived next door but one to a West Indian corner shop, which had the most unusual opening hours – for anywhere except Kilburn, that is. At 4 a.m. the shutters rolled open, and the queue half-way down the road shambled slowly in. At midnight the shutters rolled back again, and for four hours the residents of Kilburn sat waiting.

Above all, Kilburn had character – most of it bad, but unfailingly interesting.

Different areas of London had their own characteristics. Ladbroke Grove, for example, had its own rapist when I lived there and was a 'no go' area for taxis. Looking back I find it hard to believe that I would frequently walk the four miles from Paddington to home down some of the most dangerous streets in London, often in the early hours of the morning, to save 20p on the Tube. When a pint in the Middlesex Hospital students' bar cost only 16p, these things assumed an unarguable importance.

Notting Hill was a gloriously cosmopolitan area and a delight to live in, although by no means so earnestly trendy as it is now. But the area of London I loved most was Paddington, and only in Paddington could the following happen. We were sitting in the medical school canteen one Sunday afternoon when there was a tremendous crash outside, the ground literally shuddering beneath us. Paddington is not renowned for its earthquakes, nor apparently medical students for their common sense as we all immediately rushed outside to see what was going on.

Across the road, there had been a subtle change to the architecture. A charming family of Pakistanis who owned the three-storey mid-terrace newsagents had opted for a new position in the world. It collapsed in the street. Apparently the owners had decided to undertake some renovations, and sensibly enough had taken estimates from various firms. Less sensibly, they accepted a quote from a group of cowboy builders of £5,000, instead of the somewhat more realistic alternatives they had been given of around £50,000.

On Day One, the cowboy builders knocked down a supporting wall. On Day Two, the building collapsed into Praed Street. On Day Three, the builders fled the country.

I used to walk to work from Kilburn most mornings. It was cheaper than any other transport, and slower, which was always a bonus as you missed more of your lectures that way. The last leg of the journey brought you round the back of Paddington Station and along Wharf Road, so called despite the fact that it was nowhere near any wharf you could find. It did however run alongside the sort of canal you might easily fall into after a few too many in the early hours, but which no self-respecting boat would be seen within miles of.

In general the road would be pretty much empty, but on this, my inaugural day of obstetrics, the road was not empty at all. Difficult though it is to believe, whilst I was ambling down the centre of the road – universally accepted as being the safest place to walk in Paddington, at the time – I was entirely unaware of the change in the normal routine of events. Lost in thought, I managed to travel half-way though the crowds and reporters lining my route before even noticing their presence.

The explanation is simple.

For many students of the time, the morning journey to the medical school was generally spent trying (often in vain) to recollect what you had been doing the night before and how well you had been dressed whilst doing it. Hopefully you would achieve this most necessary feat of recall before anyone else chose to recollect it for you. It was essential to remember for one critical reason – so that you knew who to avoid, and for how long you should be doing it.

The crowds were cheering as I approached my destination. For one sublime moment I thought they may have congregated here as a spontaneous gesture of admiration for my succeeding in arriving before lunchtime two days in a row. I stopped, looked around, raised my arms and took their salute . . . At about the same time some chap I vaguely recognised rolled up in a Daimler from the opposite direction.

How churlish of him to spoil my one moment of adulation.

I was looking for the obstetric department, and knew it was somewhere close by. Taking advantage of this other bloke's arrival – horses, I thought absent-mindedly, something to do with horses – I slipped behind a couple of policemen and entered through the nearest door.

'Lindo Wing,' I read above it, being wholly unaware of the significance. I had only been walking past this door for the past six months or so. How was I supposed to know it was the private wing, where ladies of a certain standing came to have their babies?

Inside the noise of the crowd dimmed, and I took my bearings. For all the furore I had left behind in the street, it was remarkably quiet. After wandering the corridors aimlessly for a few minutes my destination loomed into view. 'Delivery suite', proclaimed the sign, which was precisely what I was looking for.

How was I to know it just wasn't *that* delivery suite I wanted?

Only one person seemed to notice my presence at all. 'Not a reporter?' asked a young nurse standing by reception, regarding me curiously.

'Nor am I,' I replied, moving quickly on.

If, like me, you cannot see a set of swing doors without an insatiable urge to push through them, then you, like me, would have found yourself in *that* delivery suite a few moments later.

I should remind you at this point that I had never before been in such an environment, and was uncertain as to what to expect. At first sight it looked like any other delivery suite I had seen on TV – a sweating and pain-ridden woman, an ineffectually dabbing and hand-holding husband, and me occupying Position A at the business end of the mother-to-be with a new baby whose head was just emerging into the world.

But then I began to notice one or two minor differences.

For a start, the number of people present, one of whom happened to be the Queen's gynaecologist, who had no business at all being in a delivery room with us ordinary mortals. I suddenly recalled my arrival that morning and turned my attention to the ineffectual husband I had seen stepping out of the Daimler, and beyond him a big chap immediately to my left with a bulge inside his jacket and an 'I wouldn't argue with me right now' expression on his face.

Nobody paid me the slightest attention – they were all holding their breath, waiting. I too was holding my breath and waiting, but for an entirely different reason.

Where was I? Would the statuesque giant to my left shoot me before or after the whole baby finally emerged?

With a final squeal of pain and exhilaration from the mother the baby was born, and everyone in the room – bar one – began to relax.

'It's a boy,' said the man to my left in measured tones, and then without the slightest change of expression, 'and who the bloody hell are you?'

As students we were supposed to assist the midwives at half a dozen or so births before taking the reins ourselves. Only then would we be unleashed on the unsuspecting public, on whom we should in theory complete our training by delivering – and keeping a diary of – a further twenty babies.

There are only so many babies in London to go round, so students were despatched to various parts of the country to complete their training. This was of course the ideal opportunity for the medical school to send me and a fellow inebriate, Ken, as far away from the capital as was within their capabilities.

Which is how we came to arrive in York for a two-week attachment to the obstetric unit there, neither of us as yet with any deliveries under our belts. Confidently we strode on to the wards, dreaming of babies emanating forth at regular intervals, grateful mothers sobbing their thanks and delirious fathers pressing cigars and the odd tenner into our sweating palms.

It must have been pretty nippy in York nine months previously, so indescribably perishing that every woman of child-bearing age retired to bed not just with her man but with too many layers of clothing to remove before the alarm clock went off the following morning. In addition, Yorkshire men – although being renowned for their toughness – are no doubt as lily-livered as us southerners when the prospect of frostbite in important places beneath the waist becomes a distinct possibility.

There wasn't a woman in labour to be found for miles around.

For three days and nights we sat there, gowns and gloves at the ready. For three days and nights the entire population of York failed to increase their number by a solitary figure. On the fourth day we got bored, and like all bored students our minds began to wander.

It was only a short time after that our bodies followed suit.

The only incident of any great interest occurred in the early hours of the morning, but it was entirely non-obstetric in origin. On our arrival at the hospital we were directed to our sleeping quarters, which apparently used to be barrack houses during the war. Quite interesting, really, and still with all the original furnishings. What nobody told us was that our ground-floor accommodation was next to the psychiatric wing, or I might have otherwise closed my window.

At three o'clock in the morning of the fourth day I was awoken by a tall, dishevelled man in his late forties, peering over my previously inert form.

'Where is she then?' he demanded querulously.

I felt instinctively around in the bed for a bit. Although I was pretty sure I had retired to my slumbers entirely on my own, it was evident that one complete stranger was now in my room, so why not two?

There was no one else in the bed. That was a start, and it gave me a bit of confidence.

'Who is it you are looking for?' I inquired conversationally. In retrospect, 'Who the bloody hell are you and what are you doing in my bedroom?' would have seemed a more appropriate response. It would certainly have been more in character.

'Looking for my wife, of course,' he said simply. 'I know she's in here somewhere.'

I considered carefully. I had not the least idea what was going on here, but something told me to play along, for the moment.

'Have you tried the wardrobe?' I suggested, getting into the spirit of the search. 'Or maybe behind the shower curtain?'

In truth there was more than a touch of sarcasm in this, but he took me quite literally and stepped into the adjoining bathroom while I gratefully took the opportunity to throw on my jeans and a sweater. Rubbing my eyes blearily I wandered through to join him in his search.

He was on his hands and knees in the bath, peering intently down the plug hole.

'I think I heard her calling,' he said excitedly. 'Do you think she might be stuck? Can you listen too?'

Now, no sane man that I know of would ever get in a bath at three o'clock in the morning with a complete stranger who had been looking for his wife in his bedroom, and then put his ear to the plug hole in case she should be shouting for help.

But that is exactly what I did.

It was at this point that I began to get a fit of the giggles, which once it starts I find terribly difficult to stop. There was only one thing to do. I stayed in the bath, bent over the plug hole and bit my lip viciously until I had the whole thing under control. For the first time I began to consider whether my intruder might actually be dangerous, but dismissed it out of hand.

Barking, maybe, but dangerous? Surely not . . .

This thought, which might in other circumstances be sobering, did not reduce my impending compulsion to resume giggling one iota. It was time to act.

'Sshh, I think I heard something,' I said, raising a finger to my lips. 'Look, there in the bedroom. I can see something moving.'

I dashed out of the bathroom, taking him by surprise, and made a diving leap for the window. He followed a few seconds behind me.

'She was under the bed all along,' I explained breathlessly. 'I just missed her as she was scrambling out of the window. Hurry, man, hurry. There, look, she's just going round the corner of that building. Quickly now, I'll help you out.'

I bundled him out of the window, closed it firmly in his wake and collapsed in an amorphous heap on the floor. It was only at this point that I began to wonder who he really was.

Fortunately, I did not find out for several days to come.

After three days of unutterable boredom on the delivery wards, we awoke on the fourth with a new resolve.

'All ready for work then, boys?' said the duty midwife as we strolled on to the ward. 'Another day full of opportunity awaits you.'

'It does,' I replied, 'but not in the hospital. Ken and I are off into town, to give the university the pleasure of enjoying our company.'

She looked at us dubiously. 'Old Staggers will have a fit,' she warned. 'She doesn't like her students playing hookey.'

Staggers was the name given to the consultant under whose testy eye we were supposed to be studying. She was a formidable spinster of a certain age glorying in the name of Miss Staggrington, and the consensus of opinion was that she only became an obstetrician in the hope of finally establishing for herself where babies came from.

'Old Staggers won't know,' pointed out my colleague, 'because old Staggers has gone to a meeting in Harrogate and won't be back until tomorrow morning. At least,' he added, putting on his most doleful look, 'she won't know unless somebody tells her, and you wouldn't do that to two poor culturally deprived, impoverished, terminally bored students. Would you?' He smiled beseechingly.

'We want to discover for ourselves the architectural delights of York,' I put in earnestly. 'Savour the heritage of the city, absorb the essence that is Yorkshire grit and sweat and labour . . .'

'Go to the pub,' said Ken, a look of such sheer longing washing over his cherubic features that no right-minded midwife could have failed to have her heart melted.

She raised her hands in mock defeat. 'All right, boys, your secret is safe with me. But don't, whatever you do, be late for the ward round tomorrow. I do so hate to see grown men cry.'

We tried, we really did . . .

We walked the three miles into York from the hospital, tested the local hostelries as thoroughly as time would allow and reinforced each other's firm declaration to return in time for the next day's ward round. Then we headed for the university, which to our complete surprise proved to be our undoing.

That was Thursday morning. Some time later – the following Wednesday evening, to be precise – Ken and I sat in one of the many university bars we had enjoyed to the full in the preceding week, toasting our new-found friends and acquaintances.

'Time for us to go,' said Ken solemnly. 'Now, I don't want any of you gathered here today to feel in the least bit guilty about the fact that whilst you are enjoying yourself again here tomorrow evening my colleague and I will be celebrating the end of our hopes and aspirations for the future.'

'To the end of our careers,' I said, raising my glass, and we all drank to that.

I will gloss over the events of the next morning, suffice to say that we were not greeted quite as well as the returning prodigal son. To our surprise Staggers had an unsuspected acquaintance with some of the lesser known swear words in the Yorkshire vocabulary, and I certainly learned a couple of new anatomical expressions.

That second Thursday night, the day before our departure back to the delights of London, I sat in the delivery room, contemplating what remained of my future. My first – and potentially last – delivery was finally coming to pass. The good thing about the present circumstances was that Staggers was engaged for the evening in the operating theatre with the lucky Ken, an emergency Caesarean section on her hands with two more to follow.

This jolly news was tempered by the fact that Staggers had apparently left a message on the ward to say that she would be taking a keen interest in my first delivery under her care. The innocent victim of my forthcoming attentions was to be Helen, a charming lass who had come into hospital on her own, her husband being abroad on business.

Midwives were in short supply, and at one point Helen and I were left on our own, chattering away. I confessed the sins of my past – well the past week, anyway – and she found the whole thing highly amusing.

'It might seem funny to you,' I said, 'but our consultant, Miss Staggrington, doesn't seem to see it quite the same way.'

'She can seem a bit daunting, can't she?' agreed Helen. 'But her bark is generally worse than her bite, so I understand.'

'Not if you are a derelict student,' I said, and she grinned good-humouredly.

'Well, maybe not,' she accepted. 'But I'm sure she has her good points, too.'

We sat talking for some time, waiting for something to happen. I was nervous as hell about the forthcoming delivery, and Helen, I think, was glad of the company. I did the best I could to take her mind off the fact that she was lying in labour quite on her own, with her first baby due and her family all engaged elsewhere.

She, on the other hand, was probably doing her best to forget that it was me who was going to have to deliver it.

After a while I had that nervous, twitchy feeling I used to get around twenty times a day. To my relief one of the nursing auxiliaries came in, and I stood up, stretching.

'Look,' I said, 'I'm dying for a cigarette. Would you mind if I just popped out for a moment – I'll be back in a sec.'

'Of course not,' said Helen. 'Can't keep a man from his nicotine too long, can we? I'll be fine – we'll give you a shout if we need you, won't we, nurse?'

I went outside and had my cigarette, and stopped twitching a bit – and then I had another, and stopped twitching completely. Half an hour seemed to pass before I really knew where it had gone, and as soon as I realised I made my way quickly back to the delivery suite.

As I opened the door Helen gave a shout of pain, followed by another in greeting.

'I think I'm having a baby,' she said, still smiling between gritted teeth. 'Think you could lend me a hand?'

I looked around. The delivery suite was completely empty, save for the two of us. All those days of waiting, gloves and gown at the ready, midwives on hand, obstetricians in the wings . . . and it was down to this.

Helen, myself, and a baby who would not wait.

Five minutes later it was all over.

I don't really remember much of what happened, but somehow Helen was suddenly sitting nursing a healthy eight-pound baby boy, and I am not sure which of us had the bigger smile on our face. One of the midwives came back shortly after-wards to clear up the mess I had produced – taking nearly five times longer than it had for me to create it – and I finally left.

Helen grasped my hand before I departed.

'Thanks,' she said softly. 'You were wonderful.'

'But I didn't really do anything,' I said, quite truthfully. 'It just sort of happened around me. Anyone could have done it, really.'

She smiled. 'Anyone wasn't here,' she said simply.

I lay awake for much of what remained of the night, reflecting on the vagaries of life, and the incipient meeting with Miss Staggrington the following morning. If, like a cat, a medical student has nine lives, then surely my ninth was due to come to an end in the very near future.

The following morning was the last day of our attachment. I stuck my head around Helen's door before going to the ward to discover Ken's and my fate, when to my horror I saw our executioner-to-be standing by Helen's bedside, a surprisingly benign look on her face. She peered at me over the top of her glasses.

'I've been hearing about you, young man,' she said, in what seemed intended to be a stern voice but wasn't quite succeeding.

'I've told her how wonderful you were,' Helen said, 'and how I could not have managed without you.'

'Yes, young man,' said Staggers, and to my surprise she began to smile at me. 'I think you met my favourite niece last night, did you not?'

My jaw dropped. I looked at Helen, who was beaming widely.

'You . . .' I began, and stopped. 'You . . .' I tried again. 'You didn't tell me,' I finished lamely.

She shrugged, still beaming. 'Well, you were so nervous already, I just couldn't bring myself to make it any worse for you.' She looked across at the still smiling Miss Staggrington. 'Now, you won't be cross with him any more, Auntie M, will you?'

Staggers looked at me, and I looked at her, and then Staggers looked across at Helen and the baby, sleeping peacefully in her arms.

'No,' she said slowly, 'I don't believe I will.'

Our stay in York was almost complete, but one mystery remained unexplained. Before we left, I went across to the psychiatric unit to find out who my uninvited guest had been the week before. In all the excitement of the past few days I had completely forgotten about him, for a while.

I spoke to the registrar in charge of the ward, who regarded me in an odd manner as I explained what had happened. He thought carefully for a moment or two, obviously weighing up his response, then decided to tell me.

'Oh, that was John,' he said eventually, 'and this is purely between you and me, you understand. We don't know quite how, but on the night he came to see you he had escaped from the secure unit. We were looking everywhere for him, then out of the blue he just came back with a huge smile on his face. All he would say is that he had met someone who had actually seen his wife, after all, and that it proved she was OK. He's been quiet as a mouse ever since.'

'And . . . um . . . where is his wife?' I ventured to ask, not really sure if I wanted to hear the answer.

The registrar stared back at me for a moment. 'Oh, she's dead,' he replied calmly, 'some ten years back, now. John stabbed her repeatedly, disposing of her body in a bath of lime . . .

'He's been looking for her ever since.'

51

* * *

A week later, after the so nearly ill-fated trip to York, I was back on obstetric 'duty' at the medical school. In those days the student on call used to sleep in the very same room in which Alexander Fleming discovered penicillin from the mould on his cheese sandwich, or some such thing.

I could swear the original mould was still there.

One of those tricky ethical decisions was looming. Ken and I were basking in a glowing report from York, still celebrating our fortunate escape from the probable terminal wrath of the Dean thanks to Staggers having shown a surprisingly humane side beneath her gruff exterior. Our fellow students found all this quite incomprehensible, having rightly considered it completely beyond our limited capabilities to succeed in any academic enterprise with which we were involved.

We had shed not a vestige of light on the truth that lay behind it.

'Application, dedication and sheer commitment to hard work,' I heard Ken telling some bemused colleagues.

'But you're talking about you and Sparrow!' they replied, unconvinced.

'We are changed men,' said Ken, sanctimoniously.

The horns of my current ethical dilemma were as follows. I was on call for the delivery suite, the entire West End of London relying wholly on my new-found obstetric skills, whilst my friends were poised to embark on an extended pub crawl in celebration of something or other of major importance. The end of another week, maybe; actually staying awake throughout an entire histology lecture, even when the lights went off . . . I forget the precise nature of the occasion, but a pub crawl it was.

There are essentially two types of student pub crawl. Firstly the local, which is when you simply move from one local pub to the next, secure in the knowledge that you are never too far from home to stagger back when the legs inevitably go. Secondly

– and on a grander scale – the 'special event', which generally involves a particularly difficult challenge. By far the most spectacular of these was the Circle Line, the rules of which are easily explained.

You began with a pint in the medical school bar and then headed for Paddington Station, which was the nearest underground stop to our starting point. From there you travelled around the entire Circle Line, alighting at each stop for half a pint at the nearest pub before returning back to the station you had just left, to move on to the next. You finally completed the trip – if you were still in an upright position – with a pint back in the students' hall of residence bar, just round the corner from where you had originally set out.

All very straightforward, you might think, but there were a few minor points to be taken into consideration. There are twenty-six stops on the Circle Line, which means twenty-six journeys, let alone twenty-six drinks and twenty-six sprints from the Tube station to the pub and back. Since the underground timetable had been amended a few years earlier it was now considered impossible to undertake the task in the original form the challenge had been designed – i.e. it must be entirely completed between opening time in the evening, and closing time the same night.

As far as we were aware it had never been done – which of course made it imperative that we should try. Amazingly (for medical students) this required a great deal of planning and careful forethought – amazing, because we actually managed to do it. Had we put as much effort into our studies we might all have qualified with a more than adequate knowledge of the complexities of the human body.

To prepare for the event we took a day off – not in itself an unusual occurrence – and toured the streets of London in an old Volkswagen Beetle, carefully recording the nearest pub to each station and the directions to it. Although these details would be easy to recall in the first hour or two of our attempt, it seemed likely that after twenty drinks or so the memory might dim just a little.

The final requirement was to find two volunteers to help us out. Time was precious; we had to make sure that each time we stepped off a train, we dashed to the pub and back in time for the next – miss one train and the whole affair was off. As we could not afford the time to queue for drinks, the crucial task of our volunteers was to travel ahead, each taking alternate stations and ordering our drinks in advance. We would then rush in – or progressively stagger, stumble and crawl in the latter stages of the event – down our drinks in one go, and rush off whence we came.

Looking back, I cannot think why anyone in their right mind would even begin to contemplate such lunacy. But we did, which no doubt reveals a great deal about our state of sanity at that time.

My travelling companions – who are now scattered somewhere amongst the medical profession, probably even in current day positions of great responsibility – were Neil Moat and Tez McCormack, who I believe later became one of the Teletubbies. I cannot recall for certain who the third of our party was, but I think it was Biffo the Bear – aka Dr Michael Lacey.

All we needed now was the right day for the task, and providence soon shone upon us. On 1st April 1977 the underground station staff and ticket collectors went on strike, refusing to collect any fees. The entire journey could be done for free . . .

After a week's hard training, running from pub to pub and drinking too much – tough work, but all in a good cause – we were ready. We started at 5 o' clock in the medical school bar, downed our first pint and set off on the seemingly unattainable.

History records – but my memory does not – that we returned, task duly completed, at 10.15 p.m. No cheating, no throwing up and no ability to remain vertical for more than a few moments at a time. It remains one of the highlights of our quiet, studious medical careers.

Another, but less physically demanding, 'special event' crawl was the five-legged race around ten pubs in Paddington. Teams of three – two men, one woman, legs duly tied together – had to complete a set course, a pint in each pub for the men, a short of their choice for the women. The winner was the first team home, in the unlikely event that anyone made it home at all.

My male partner that day was a fellow student by the name of Dave Langford. I believe he once attended a lecture in the first year, but that may just be a vicious rumour. Unfortunately our prospective female counterpart, the cog in an as yet unlubricated wheel, had sensibly found something better to do, and failed to turn up.

True, it may be that she considered anything at all would be better than being trussed inescapably between Mr Langford and myself, but we felt signally let down. Whilst I was considering how to exhibit my extreme hurt and the resultant severe psychological setback, the good Mr Langford was doing something about it – namely, chatting up every unattached (literally) female in the bar. The major hurdle that seemed initially insuperable was that each such female present knew the pair of us well, and had far more sense than to be roped in on the occasion.

However, as luck would have it – most definitely ours, and not hers at all – Louisa, an American medical student who had landed in the country only a matter of hours previously, wandered at that precise moment into the bar. This was no doubt a mistake she would regret for many years to come, as Dave moved in for the Langford charm offensive.

Minutes later Louisa was firmly and inescapably ensconced between the pair of us. It seemed little in the way of a hindrance at the time that she was extremely pretty.

'How lucky you are,' I lied comprehensively, 'to have joined us at such an auspicious moment.'

'Are we likely to win?' she asked innocently.

'Not a chance,' I said firmly. 'Unless . . . what we need is an edge.'

Dave's face lit up in a demonic grin. 'I know,' he said. 'We'll drive.'

'We cannot drive,' I told him, and for a moment I meant it. 'This is a five-legged pub crawl, not a five-legged and a car pub crawl.'

'It's not against the rules,' he persisted.

'There are no rules,' I replied.

'Precisely. That's my point.'

I gave it one last shot. 'It's against the law. It's morally reprehensible. We might spill our drinks . . .' I lapsed into silence.

'We'll win,' he said emphatically.

We drove.

Or at least Dave drove, our American friend sat uncomfortably astride the gear lever of his MG and I occupied the passenger seat. We were supremely confident, secure in the knowledge that we were doing it in style.

Between the third and fourth pub, we were arrested. I will not easily forget the look on the face of the young policeman as he flagged down our car, beckoning us to disembark.

'Would you hold my pint?' asked David, handing it to Louisa with an innocent air that Gandhi himself would have been proud of.

He stepped out of the car, dragging Louisa behind him and I followed, in part resignation and part relief that I had no car of my own.

Spare a thought, as I suspect we did not, for our poor American colleague. Barely an hour and a half into her putative English medical career and she was arrested tied between two complete strangers, charming and debonair though they may have been, following which she was incarcerated in a cell in Paddington Green Police Station.

I did not attend the court.

Nor, for that matter, did Louisa, who had caught the first plane back to Virginia following our release. Strangely, there were no more visiting American students for some time.

The good Mr Langford strolled into the bar a month later, grinning from ear to ear.

'They let me off,' he said several pints later when he eventually stopped for a breather, 'with a warning. They said they had never heard anything like it, and that initiative should be encouraged. "Students will be students," said the one in the middle, "but some will be more students than others," and then they all burst out laughing.'

Memories of these glorious days flooded back to me as I sat in Fleming's room of inadvertent discovery. The horns of my dilemma, once now deliberated upon, were soon addressed. I wandered down to the ward at around seven o'clock in the evening, and casually asked, 'Anything happening?'

'Oh, yes,' answered the midwife on duty, looking at her watch. 'The kettle's boiling, Sister Jensen has just gone to the loo, the lady in bed three is complaining about her piles, and *Emmerdale Farm* is starting in less than a minute.'

Mary's does this to you – you enter, full of enthusiasm, dedicated to your lifelong calling, and before you know it, flippancy takes over.

'I was thinking in terms of women in labour,' I said, trying not all that successfully to stand on my dignity.

She regarded me with interest. 'Excuse me?' she said. 'Have I made a mistake here? You are the same student who told Professor Beard' (head of the obstetric department) 'that the reason you didn't attend his lecture was because you felt unworthy of sitting in the same room as him?'

I nodded.

'And you are the same student who said that a woman in labour had just joined the wrong political party?'

I nodded again.

'And you are looking for something to do?' she finished incredulously.

'Not . . . entirely,' I answered. 'Just thought I might . . .'

'Nip out for a drink?' she suggested.

'Nip out for a drink,' I agreed.

'So predictable,' she sighed, 'and so unlikely to succeed.'

I must have looked genuinely hurt, because she leaned forward and rested her hand on my shoulder.

'Sorry, Mike, but if everybody says it, it must be true. I wouldn't want to hide anything from you.'

'Well, are you currently hiding any women in labour?' I inquired.

'None,' she relented. 'Go and have a drink with your friends. Just make a half-way passable attempt to come back sometime this decade.'

'I'll ring,' I called happily over my shoulder, 'around nine o'clock.'

Well, midnight is around nine o'clock, just not closely around, if you must be pedantic. There was still nothing happening, on the labour ward at least, but out on the mean streets of Paddington things were beginning to roll.

I decided to roll with them.

At three o'clock in the morning what remained of our entourage sat in the Ring O'Bells, less than a hundred yards from the hospital. Well, I was within reach, I consoled myself, in case of an emergency.

The telephone rang.

'That'll be for me,' I said confidently, and lifted the receiver before the appalled landlord could prevent me.

'This is the police,' came a clipped voice. 'Listen carefully. You are about to be raided, ten minutes at most. I suggest you move fast.' The line went dead.

An interesting approach to law enforcement, in those days. Interesting, but amazingly effective. I passed on the good news to our host, who took it calmly.

'OK, boys, Plan A,' he snapped, moving fast.

'What's Plan B?' asked Neil, my flatmate, curiously.

'Never needed one, Neil,' he threw back, lifting the till and fleeing upstairs. 'Plan A works every time.'

And in truth, Plan A was simple, but effective. It went like this.

The publican and his wife ran upstairs, turned the lights off and pretended to be asleep. The publican's paying – and consequently illegal – guests, in other words ourselves, fled across the road and round the corner, peering out from behind the pornographic book-shop, and watched the fun.

Sure enough, five minutes later a fleet of police cars screamed to a halt outside the Ring O'Bells and vomited forth their occupants, who began battering on the door. A bleary-eyed landlord, clad only in his dressing gown, opened the door and professed his completely unconvincing disgust at being disturbed at such an unearthly hour in the morning.

This long-rehearsed pantomime having been duly played out, those of us who were still able to do so watched the police cars roar off and then crossed the road and re-entered the pub. The till was already back in its rightful place, our glasses were replen-ished and off we went again, until dawn broke and the party broke with it.

I awoke the next morning, wondering, as one does on such occasions, where I was and what precisely I was doing there, and when my eyes eventually focused on the good Dr Fleming's long-established mould, realisation finally hit home. 'Thank God,' I said to myself, 'there were no deliveries on the ward last night.'

'Thank God,' I repeated to the duty sister shortly afterwards, 'there were no deliveries on the ward last night.'

She raised an eyebrow. 'Thank God,' she said slowly, 'I am never likely to be one of your patients.'

There was a message here somewhere, and I was beginning to receive it.

'Those whom the gods seek to destroy,' she continued, 'they send first to Mary's when you are on duty.'

I must have looked almost as humble as I felt, and she relented a little.

'Bed number six,' she revealed, 'and start crawling when you get to bed number four.'

I decided to brazen it out, and make no mention of my precursory visit to the pub – well, numerous pubs – the previous evening.

As I approached bed number six, where a large, jovial-looking lady sat surrounded by flowers, chocolates and innumerable children of various denominations, my resolution dissolved completely.

'Was I very drunk?' I asked simply.

She nodded slowly. 'Very,' she admitted. 'I particularly enjoyed the part where you tried to put your gown on upside down. I particularly enjoyed it because you actually succeeded in doing it.'

A huge grin spread across her face.

Looks are not everything. I fell in love with her that second.

'But I didn't enjoy that quite as much as when you – '

'Stop,' I pleaded. 'Please stop. I apologise for everything.'

She looked around her at the gaggle of children all pressing for a sight of her latest born.

'I had eight children when I came in here last night', she said. 'Eight labours, all different, all in varying degrees of pain, solitude, silence and discomfort. But in only one labour – yours – have I laughed so much and enjoyed myself so unreservedly. There, take a look at her. She's beautiful.'

She handed me a small bundle of blankets, and the most perfect baby I had ever seen peered shyly out at me. My heart melted.

'I've called her after you,' she said softly.

Michaela Hopkins, wherever you may be, I love your mother still.

4

A Trip to South Africa

It was another glorious day at the office.

I awoke. The hospital was beckoning, my patients were in need of me, my vocation was calling . . . but on the other hand, the sun was shining, the sky azure blue . . .

So I went to the beach.

For this was Cape Town, January 1978, and I was here on my 'elective'.

Somewhere during the third or fourth year of medical school every student has a three-month spell when they can elect – hence the term 'elective' – to work at any hospital of their choice. For those with their eyes on a high-flying career this may well mean staying at their own hospital to work with one of the eminent professors or consultants, hoping to secure a post in their team following qualification.

Some will opt for a spell in another hospital in the UK. This may be because of a particular medical interest, perhaps it might just be closer to home, or else they are simply really boring people without the inclination to travel.

But for the rest of us it is a chance to escape the confines of London and travel to a destination of our choice. I had friends who went to Australia, South America, Brighton . . . but for me it had to be Cape Town, a place I had always wanted to visit.

Politically naïve though I was, I knew that trouble was brewing in South Africa. However, this might be my only chance to go there, so despite reservations from my family I booked my flight and waited impatiently for the day of departure to arrive.

And so here I was, lying on the beach on my second morning in the country, undoubtedly the whitest Caucasian on view anywhere in sight. Everywhere I went people would point at me, whispering behind their newspapers as I passed.

To get on in this world you have to be dedicated, and to be honest, tanning does not come easily to a reddish-haired Midlander ('No, you haven't got red hair, you're ginger!' exclaimed my other half on reading this for the first time) with a sensitive skin. You have to work at it, throw yourself into it big time, prepare yourself mentally to sweat it out on that golden stretch of sand just a few hours longer, no matter how much it may hurt, no matter what the sacrifices you must make.

And it can be tough. You have to take your own towel, search for that one spot all the really good-looking women will stroll past on a regular basis and remember precisely when the bar opens, and when it is going to close.

I had arrived in Cape Town unexpectedly. That is, unexpected by them, but not by me as I knew where I was going when I bought the ticket. Finally, after a few interesting moments en route, there I was, standing in the office of the Dean's secretary on a Friday morning while she was wondering what on earth she was going to do with me. I can no longer remember her surname, but her smile and her Christian name will be etched on my heart for as long as I live.

Never has the name Susan seemed so bewitching, either before or since.

'Hi,' she said, beaming at me as if we had just met on a blind date. 'I'm Susan, I'm the Dean's secretary, and I have not the least idea what you are doing in my office unless you have mistaken it for the shower room you so obviously need, and whilst we are on the subject – which I suppose you could argue we are not, as yet – I really do not like your shirt. How may I help you?'

'You don't like my shirt?' I asked pitifully. 'I've travelled by foot, bus, train, aeroplane, camel, bicycle, taxi, tram and Chinese junk over the last two weeks, and eaten more than one British Rail sandwich. I've been spat upon, mugged, beaten up, deified, anointed by maverick Hebrews as an alternative saviour, survived an entire night at the YMCA in Johannesburg and yet despite all that I have made my way here, bloodied but unbowed, my favourite shirt upon my back . . . And you ask how you can help me, and say you don't like my shirt! How much more can one man be expected to go through in the furtherance of his chosen vocation? How much, I ask you?'

She regarded me steadily for a moment, and then sighed gently. 'Of course,' she said finally, 'you're English, aren't you?'

'Yes,' I admitted.

'Then that explains everything,' she shrugged, before adding shrewdly 'Do you actually know where you are?'

I nodded. 'Eight hours thirty-five minutes from Heathrow.'

'So's Luton,' she said, a smile twitching at the corners of her mouth, 'if you go by the M25.'

I grinned.

'Well,' she continued after a moment, obviously deciding that standing and grinning were the only two useful contributions I had to make to proceedings, 'why are you here, exactly?'

'Why are any of us here?' I countered.

She tried again. 'What is it that you want?'

'Oh,' I considered, 'what do any of us want? A rich and fulfilling life, someone to hold on to at night, children, a Volvo, maybe a fortnight in Lanzarote every now and then – it's the simple things, don't you think, that make life so worth the living?'

She smiled, despite herself, and reached across her desk for the telephone. 'Well, it's been nice talking to you,' she said. 'Unusual, but nice. So if you don't mind, I'll be getting on with the rest of my life now – can you find your own way out, or would you like to wait till security get here to show you? Security are very big,' she added thoughtfully, 'and inclined to random acts of wanton violence.'

'Depends how long they take,' I said, considering, and then I gave up. 'Oh, I give up. I'm here on elective, from England, and I'm tired, I'm hungry, I'm not all that clean, and it would be ever so nice if you could help me find a way to attend to all three.'

She frowned, furrowing her brow, which made her look even prettier than before, if that were possible.

'Elective . . . England . . . that sort of rings a bell, somehow,' she said, and putting the phone down she crossed to a filing cabinet by the door, passing in front of me. She smelled as fragrant as I did unsavoury – in other words very fragrant indeed.

A few moments of concerted rummaging later and she emerged with a small folder. Opening it, she slowly turned the pages before stopping at one, running her finger down a column of names until it came to a halt, tapping the page.

'Sparrow, Michael,' she read, looking up at me. 'That's you, is it?'

'Unfortunately,' I agreed. 'So I am in the right country, then?'

'At the moment, yes,' she replied, 'but we have a really efficient deportation process – I'll alert them to your presence first thing in the morning. Now, where are you staying?'

'Staying?' I repeated, surprised.

'Yes, staying – as in where are you intending to live whilst we are enduring your presence?' But she was smiling as she said it.

'Well, I was hoping for somewhere with walls, a roof, doors and stuff.'

'No, I'm being serious,' she said, suddenly concerned. 'Do you not actually have anywhere to stay?'

'No, I don't,' I admitted with a sigh. 'I sort of had this vague idea that the medical school might have arranged it.'

'And I suppose you still believe in the Tooth Fairy and Father Christmas?'

'Doesn't everyone?' I asked in mock surprise.

She looked at me. 'I think,' she said slowly, curling her lip delectably, 'that someone is going to have to take you in hand.'

'Someone?' I mused.

'Someone,' she repeated, smiling broadly, 'and as I seem to be the only someone around here at the moment . . .'

She picked up the phone again and dialled quickly. 'Hi, Brenda, it's Susan,' she said after a voice spoke at the other end. 'You remember when you said anyone would do? Did you mean it, because I think I've got anyone here in my office at the moment.'

I could hear laughter at the other end of the line, and then Susan said, 'I'll send him right over. His name is Michael, and I'd start running the bath and opening all the windows, if I were you.'

'Are your friends particularly dirty, then?' I asked innocently.

'Stop it,' she said, 'I have work to do. Look, my brother, Simon, is a medical student too, and he left for England on *his* elective the day before yesterday. He shares a house with some friends of mine, and they're looking for someone to rent his room for three months or so. Will that do, do you think?'

'That will do perfectly,' I said, relieved. 'Is it far?'

She beckoned me over to the window, and pointed. 'All the way down that hill,' she said, pointing to a small bungalow gleaming brilliant white in the sunshine no more than a couple of hundred yards away. 'Do you think you can make it?'

'I think I can make it,' I promised. 'What should I do when I get there?'

She stood and regarded me carefully, her long blonde hair catching the light. 'Apologise,' she said finally, 'and then come back here tomorrow morning, nine o'clock sharp, with any shirt you may have other than this one. Should be safe enough – the Dean never gets here until at least nine thirty at the weekend. I'll have to break you in gently . . .'

I made my way down the hill from the hospital a good deal more easily than I had made my way up, wondering if Susan could possibly have been as perfect as she seemed and reflecting it was pretty unlikely that I would ever find out. The door of the bungalow was open, and I knocked tentatively, calling, 'Hello? Anyone in?'

And that's when I met Brenda and Linda.

Brenda and Linda were identical twins, which is a bit like saying you cannot tell the difference between an orange and a banana. Linda was tall, large-boned and curly-haired, whereas Brenda was a sort of concertinaed version – short, round and curly-haired. They assured me as we got to know each other better that they really were identical but that Linda had helped herself to a few of Brenda's genes in utero, and Brenda had a really healthy appetite.

They welcomed me in and I felt immediately at home.

'There's a cat on your bed,' said Brenda. 'We thought about moving it, but decided that from what Susan was saying it was probably cleaner than you were. So we just left it and ran the bath instead. Is that OK?'

'That's just perfect,' I said thankfully. 'It's been a very long journey.'

'And not a very clean one,' put in Linda, 'by the look of it.'

'Well,' I admitted, 'there was no bath on the train, and quite frankly although I stayed at the YMCA in Johannesburg, it wasn't a place where I felt comfortable about taking any of my clothes off.'

'Very wise,' agreed Brenda – they seemed to take it in turns to speak, 'but definitely not a policy to be continued in Cape Town, if you want to be living here throughout your stay. Coffee's on – would you like some?'

Ten minutes later I was lying in a steaming hot bath, a mug of coffee in my hand. The January sun was pouring in through a window through which I could see Table Mountain rising majestically above the hospital, Groote Schuur, and I remember thinking God had indeed smiled upon me for a while.

I intended to make the most of it.

The following morning I was back inside the office with Susan, and very nearly at the time she had suggested, as well. She was of course there ahead of me, looking even more radiant than she had the day before.

She looked up as I came in and did an elegant double-take. 'My,' she said approvingly, 'don't you brush up well.'

'Occasionally,' I admitted, 'but it takes a hell of a lot of brushing.'

'Grab a seat,' she pointed, opening a drawer in her desk. 'I have something for you.'

'Oh goody,' I said. 'Is it sweets and biscuits?'

She stopped rummaging for a second, and frowned, which she did as beautifully as everything else, all the more so because she was totally unaware of it. 'Do people get exasperated with you a lot?'

'Quite a lot.'

'It figures.' She shrugged, and then smiled again. 'But I suppose you'll only be here for three months. I guess I . . . I guess we can cope with you for that long, if we all pull together. And anyway, this should help a bit.'

She handed across a piece of paper embossed with the hospital logo, and I read it at first uncomprehendingly.

'This is to confirm,' it said, 'that Michael Sparrow has duly completed his three-month elective at Groote Schuur Hospital with the highest commendation,' and at the foot of the sheet, below the Dean's signature, was a date three months hence.

'But this is . . . I haven't . . . surely you can't . . .' I burbled. 'How did you get him to . . . ?' I ground pathetically to a halt. 'It's not April Fool's Day, is it?'

She reached forward and gently took the piece of paper from my hand, regarding it with a contemplative eye. 'You know,' she said, reflecting, 'I'm getting better and better at his signature each time I try it.'

Realisation struck me like a thunderbolt. 'You mean you . . . ?'

'Yes, me,' she said, staring at me so hard I began to perspire from places I didn't yet know the correct anatomical phraseology for. 'Call me stupid, but somehow I have begun to form the impression that you, work and hospitals are a totally mismatched trio. And besides . . .' and for a fleeting moment a hint of shyness flitted across her face, 'I'm on holiday for a fortnight, starting tomorrow. Won't you be needing someone to show you around?'

I loved South Africa.

For a young medical student who had never before been abroad it was an eye-opener of tremendous proportions. Unlike many people, I have never been given to take any interest in the country I am travelling to prior to departure, preferring to take each experience as it comes, so although I was vaguely aware of apartheid – some boring political stuff that bloke Peter Hain was forever rabbiting on about – I had little or no idea of what it actually meant. All it took was a critically full bladder at Johannesburg airport to strike the first note of reality into my blissfully naïve savoir faire.

I looked around the bustling terminal and with heartfelt relief at last spotted the sign I was so desperately seeking – a male outline with a small notice beneath it saying 'Coloured'. I needed the loo, and I needed it now.

I was just walking through the entrance when a large man with a bullet-shaped head clasped me firmly on the shoulder and said harshly 'You can't go in there, mate.'

'I can,' I said mildly. 'Just watch – one foot in front of the other, and before you know it, there I will be. Try it with me, if you like – don't worry, you'll be fine. I'll talk you through the whole thing.'

'I said, "You can't go in there,"' he repeated menacingly, pointing to the sign. 'Look, it says coloured.'

'I don't care what colour it is,' I responded sweetly. 'Green would be nice, or maybe a pretty pastel pink, but the way my bladder is feeling I would be happy with a slightly stained beige, or even a bit of grey.'

'You go there,' he grunted, spinning me round and pushing me in the direction of a second entrance I had not previously noticed. 'In there, everything is white, just like you and me. Got the picture?'

And I had, belatedly.

At first I couldn't get to grips with it at all. Take bars, for example. Some men – and I freely admit that I am one – are brought up to lean, sprawl and then finally slump upon them until closing time or unconsciousness is upon us, whichever should arrive first. A bar stool, a pint, a cigarette and a packet of pork scratchings, and all is right in the world.

But you couldn't lean on a bar in Johannesburg, or Cape Town. You were supposed to sit at a table and click your fingers, at which point a coloured waiter would come, take your order and return with your drink. All the white people sitting, all the coloured and black waiting upon them.

No matter how hard I tried, I couldn't get used to it.

'I just want to order my own drink, and carry it myself to wherever I want to sit,' I would try to explain unsuccessfully, but eventually I would have to succumb to the inevitable. How long, I began to wonder, before I too began to sit and click impatiently, along with rest of them?

I have scattered memories of South Africa.

Running each day up the footpaths to the Cecil Rhodes monument on Table Mountain, wandering the streets of Cape Town blithely ignorant of the dangers . . .

'You mean you went *there?*' Brenda or Linda would say, aghast. 'Are you *mad?*'

I was busy developing a tan to be proud of, day after day of lying on the beach. Occasionally, however, when the weather was bad I would turn up for work, instead. Groote Schuur was where Christian Barnard had been transplanting hearts for the first time, or so we were all led to believe.

'Spent all his time at news conferences telling the rest of the world how clever he was,' said a registrar bitterly to me one day, 'while the rest of us were actually getting on with the work.' But what stays indelibly in my mind is the tragedy of the oil drum victims.

Out there, as in so many strife-torn countries I have visited in later years, it was the inter-tribal warfare that was the worst of all. So many things were done to so many people in the cause, but there was one particularly macabre vengeance that was wreaked upon rival gang members.

The first time I saw this I just stood, unable to believe my eyes. A young boy, no more than seventeen, was tied around the circumference of an oil drum, head lolling to one side, eyes open, expressionless.

'What – ' I began, taking a step forward, only to stop as Craig, a South African registrar, took firm hold of my arm.

'Wait,' he said tersely. 'We have to make sure he's not booby-trapped, first.'

We were outside the hospital in the car park, late at night, in response to a phone call a few minutes earlier. 'Come on,' said Craig. 'Part of your education. Come on and see what the locals do to each other as part of a fun Saturday night out.'

'Is he . . . he's not dead, is he?' I asked, staring at the lifeless body in front of us.

'Oh no,' said Craig grimly. 'It's worse than that. They tie them round the barrel and stick fine needles in the back of their necks – their knowledge of anatomy is probably as good as yours or mine – and wiggle those needles about until they've done as much damage to the spinal cord as they can without killing them. Make a few mistakes along the way, of course, but they're getting pretty good at it by now.'

He bent over the inert body. 'This one – dead from the neck down, I would say, but they've overdone it. Can't see him lasting until morning. One of their failures, thank God for him.'

'And what's a success, for goodness sake?' I wondered out loud.

'Dead from the neck down, but alive enough to survive and be fully aware of what's happened to them. The closest thing to a living hell I've ever come across. Come on, he's safe enough. Give me a hand – we'd better get him inside for what's left of the night.'

Not all was doom and gloom during my stay, though – in fact, far from it. Linda and Brenda looked after me wonderfully well, and although I have never seen them since I left I remember their kindness with great affection.

Brenda was a pharmacist, and worked in the hospital dispensary. One of her jobs was to make up what we used to call 'Brompton Cocktails', a morphine-based concoction which acted as a strong painkiller for terminally ill patients. In those days it would have a variety of long since banned ingredients including cocaine, which is still used intermittently as a local anaesthetic.

'We have this big pot of it,' she explained one day, a mischievous look on her face. 'It comes as a powder, and nobody ever checks it, so I dispense it by the tablespoon. One for the patient, one for me . . .'

I was never quite sure if she was serious.

More importantly Susan had an uncle who owned a vineyard at Stellenbosch, and she kindly took me out for a visit. Even more kindly she left me there and came back to pick me up three days later, which showed just what a splendid woman she was.

Most of the day – or at least, the bit that did not involve testing the produce – was spent wandering among the vines with Harry, Susan's uncle, a couple of Rottweilers and one of the house boys, who rejoiced in the name of Chocolate Box. Another went by the name of Bedsprings, which I thought a touch unusual until

Harry explained that one of the local customs was to name the newborn child after the first thing they would probably have seen on their entry into the world.

'Doesn't apply to breech births, of course,' said Harry solemnly before snorting loudly and collapsing into gales of laughter.

Susan and I were getting along famously. This was in part because she was great fun and remarkably tolerant, and also because I had yet to blot my copy-book irrevocably – an unusual state of affairs given the amount of time I had been in the country.

It was obviously time for the Big Test – in other words what you expose your relationship to before it becomes one of those 'I missed you and I bought you a present' sort of things.

South Africans, then as now, loved their sport. When I was there they were suffering from the ban on international competition, and the most important sporting event of them all was the interstate rugby cup. The final was to be held in Cape Town during my stay, and not only did I have a ticket but also an invitation to a post-match party hosted by friends of Susan's parents.

It was confidently anticipated that I would be on my best behaviour there . . . And I tried, I really did.

I went to the game with Porsche, a geology student I had come to know well after a particularly riotous evening in one of the local bars. 'No, it's not because I was born in one,' he explained about his name, 'I just always wanted to own one, and this is the closest I ever got.' He and I, together with a couple of his friends, had a few drinks in the bar before the game, a couple or so at half-time, and just one or two more after the match had finished.

At this point in the proceedings the woman behind the bar began to look exceedingly attractive, and when I repaired there for the next round of drinks she asked with a knowing smile if I would like to meet her round the back after her shift was due to finish. Duly flattered, but of course not in the least bit interested,

I confided as much to Porsche in a man-to-man sort of way when I returned to my seat.

He patted me on the arm sympathetically, turned to his friends and announced in a loud voice, 'Hey, the doc's on a promise from Alicia,' and they all started laughing.

'Am I missing something here?' I ventured to ask, and they all laughed quite a lot more. 'Am I missing something important?'

'Yes,' said Porsche emphatically, and 'Yes,' said his friends in unison, and 'Yes,' shouted everyone else in the bar, including Alicia, smiling broadly.

And then the awful truth struck home. 'She's a man, isn't she?' I said faintly.

South African parties had a strange custom which I did not at first appreciate. You took your own meat and drink, whilst the hosts supplied the venue, the salad, the cooking facilities and the hopefully attractive members of the opposite sex.

Porsche, whose brother was a butcher, had kindly provided steak for us all and had some cans of beer in the car. And this is where the Big Test began to form . . . I decided to take a bottle of whisky, a drink I am not especially fond of, intending to share it in return for the odd can or two.

We drove to the party which was in one of the smartest areas of Cape Town. Still that sense of foreboding, of impending doom that by now I should have been so fully aware of, continued to elude me. The place was packed, and it was a good twenty minutes before I finally bumped into Susan, who looked bewitching in a white dress.

'You're getting drunk, aren't you,' she said thoughtfully. I nodded.

'Thought so,' she continued, adding 'Do you think I'm going to need to pretend I've never met you before a bit later on?'

'Almost certainly,' I agreed. 'Maybe best to start doing that now.'

'OK,' she said happily, giving me a kiss on the cheek, 'and

then we could pretend to meet for the first time again, couldn't we, and . . .' She whispered in my ear, and not for the first time I wondered if it was possible to improve upon perfection.

My downfall, I am convinced, was due solely to the shortage of glasses. The bottle of whisky I had in my pocket surely played no part in it . . . but maybe I am deluding myself. Porsche took a deep breath, plunged into the crowd and returned triumphantly a few minutes later with two pint glasses.

'Last two in the place,' he said, cracking a can and emptying it into his glass. I opened the bottle of whisky, talking away, and looked down a second or two later to find I had inadvertently filled the glass to the brim. There was no way I was going to manage to pour it back, in that crowd. I started to mingle.

There is a moment, clearly imprinted upon my memory, when I recall looking down at the glass in my hand and noticing with at first curiosity, next astonishment, then rapidly following each other alarm and finally abject panic that the glass was empty. More worryingly, I was pretty sure I had not spilt any.

That elusive sense of foreboding was becoming less elusive by the second.

It was like the eye of the storm, the still before dawn, the moment when you know that something unutterably awful is about to happen and you are powerless to prevent it. That moment was upon me now.

I was standing with my back to a glass table on which all the food had been carefully laid out, when a very curious thing happened. It was something so bizarre and surreal that I found myself unable to move for a while, stunned by the sheer unexpectedness of events and the speed of my fall from the plateau of grim reality to the paranormal abyss opening up beneath my feet . . .

The table had risen vertically, thrown itself at my back and smashed in half, hurling plates, cutlery, salad bowls and all manner of meat and vegetables up into the air in a huge glassy maelstrom, with me at its centre. So amazed was I by this remarkable feat of anti-gravity I did not at first comprehend why I was lying flat on my back on the floor, surrounded by the wreckage of what but a few moments ago had been the entire company's much anticipated dinner, with the assembled crowd looking down at me in a state of shock.

By a second feat of anti-gravity even more remarkable than the first, I rose to my feet and headed for the door before anything worse could happen – were that in any way within the bounds of possibility – and out into the street, and oblivion . . .

'He's alive, then,' I could hear Porsche saying somewhere far in the distance. I opened my eyes slowly with that 'Oh my God, where am I and how on earth did I get here?' feeling I once used to know so well.

Porsche, Brenda, Linda, Susan and a couple of interested bystanders were gathered at the door of the room. I began to focus vaguely on my surroundings, realising I was somehow back in my own bed, which was almost the last place anyone, including myself, would have expected to find me.

Susan sighed heavily and walked across to where I lay, pathetically ashamed of myself despite my complete inability at that stage to recall what it was I had to be ashamed of. There are some times when you just know . . .

She sat down on the edge of the bed and gave me one of those looks.

'I don't know whether to kick you or hug you,' she said. 'Run away as fast as I can or crawl in beside you until you regain some sort of consciousness. How you ever made it four miles across town given the state you were in defeats me completely – we followed you out into the street but you had vanished without trace. God knows where you've bloody well been, you horrible, horrible man you. You've had us all worried to death, damn you, looking all over the place for you and all the time you've been lying here sleeping it off you . . . you . . .'

She ground to a halt, speechless for a second or two.

'One day,' she continued at last, 'just maybe one day we will be able to look back at this and all of us laugh and think how funny it was. But that day is not today, and won't be tomorrow, either.'

And then her expression softened perceptibly, and she bent over and kissed me gently on the forehead. 'But I'm so glad you're safe, damn you to hell and back,' she said, and standing up she turned and walked away, out of the room.

I lay there, all sorts of thoughts flooding through my mind.

'I wish,' I murmured under my breath, 'I hadn't done that. I really wish I hadn't done that at all.'

My stay in South Africa was intended to be only three months, but once I was there, and the sun was shining, it seemed such a shame to be going home. I decided to extend my visit and face the music on my return . . .

At the end of my sojourn in Cape Town I flew back to Johannesburg and took a train via Pretoria up to Petersburg, where an old school friend of my mother's was living. She had married a South African Boer, and I looked forward to a fortnight's leisurely rest before returning to Britain.

Sadly, things did not work out as planned.

Jean, my mother's friend, was delightful, but her husband Frank was probably the most bigoted, unpleasant individual I had ever met. After the gentle tolerance of most people I had encountered in Cape Town this came as a disagreeable surprise.

He was one of the officials in charge of the local black township, and the day after my arrival took me for a tour of the area. I had seen some of the poverty and deprivation in the country during my stay, but nothing had prepared me for the desolation of the shanty towns we were seeing.

Yet it was Frank's overbearing attitude that disturbed me the most.

'There's just no point in building them decent houses,' he told me as we travelled around the tents and corrugated shelters in which the local inhabitants were somehow scratching a living in. 'Give them a wooden door and they'll rip it off to use it for firewood.' He turned to look at me with an expression of disgust on his face.

'You can take the Kaffir' (a derogatory term the white population sometimes used for the black) 'out of the jungle,' he said harshly, 'but you can never take the jungle out of the Kaffir.'

I left after two days, unable to stand it any longer.

5

Arrival on the Wards

Exams were all over.

I had qualified at last, found myself a job, taken a short holiday, and set off on the first leg of my new career. I was a doctor, I had letters after my name, I was ready for anything . . .

In fact, I was terrified.

And then suddenly there I was, arriving on my first ward as a junior houseman, the most inexperienced doctor in the hospital. It was Friday, 4 p.m., and the weekend loomed ominously before me. The Senior House Officer (SHO) – qualified for two years and on a par with God's elder brother, to my innocent eyes – greeted me rapturously.

'How nice to see you,' he enthused warmly. I felt immediately valued, part of the team, an essential cog in the smooth running of the well-oiled machine that is our vocation. I was a doctor at last. I felt important. I was needed.

'Thought I was stuck here for the weekend,' he went on. 'Wasn't expecting you till Monday. I'm Shaheed, this is the ward, those...' pointing vaguely to the office, 'are the nurses, these sick-looking people in the flat white things with sheets on are the patients, and now that you have arrived I'm going off duty.'

And then he was gone, just as I was about to pretend I was the third-choice plumber who had come to give an over-inflated quote for the blocked sink in side ward three.

I have not, as yet, seen a sick parrot. But boy, can I sympathise.

There is a hierarchy in the world of medicine that most people think they understand. At the top is God. You know him as the consultant – leaps tall buildings in a single bound, knows what all the blades in a Swiss Army knife are for and once gave the Queen's second cousin an enema.

Below him, the Senior Registrar. Then the Junior Registrar, the Senior Senior House Officer, the Junior Senior House Officer and finally the bloke straight out of medical school who can just about tie his own shoelaces but we all know he only learned that last Thursday. That is . . . me.

But you're wrong. It's not that way at all.

I looked around and decided to go to the top. Head for the person with the real power. I went to the cleaner, and asked her what I should do next.

She pointed me towards the nurses' station – the meeting point on the ward for all nurses between tea breaks and bedpan emptying – and I walked across tentatively to be confronted by a tall, rather forbidding-looking Nigerian sister with impeccable cheekbones and an imperious nose.

She glanced down the latter at me. 'I'm Sister Whitehead,' she introduced herself.

'Hello,' I replied nervously.

'And I suppose you must be the new houseman,' she added dubiously.

'I suppose I must be,' I replied, 'because it says so on this name tag they handed me when I arrived. I just don't really feel like a doctor, that's all.'

'You don't look much like one, either,' she agreed, 'but I suppose you'll have to do. I have seen worse,' she continued encouragingly, 'but . . .'

Great start, I thought, but then she smiled warmly and I began to relax. She was human after all, and had a reassuring air about her.

'Right,' she said briskly, 'a few bits of paperwork for you, and then I'll show you around the ward. There are twenty-six patients here, and Mr Walpole will expect you to know about all of them when he gets back on Monday.'

'He's not actually here, then?' I asked naïvely.

She gave me a pitying look. 'He's a consultant, my dear boy. There are only two things he is interested in at weekends – his private patients and his golf, but not necessarily in that order.'

'So . . . who is here, then, apart from me?' I was beginning to panic. 'Shaheed's just gone – is there a registrar, or . . .'

She was shaking her head soberly. 'No, no registrar. No SHO. In fact – no anybody. Just you. You are it. But we are not on call this weekend, so there's no need to worry. Much.'

'And if I need some help?' I stuttered pathetically. 'What if . . . I mean when . . .' I tailed off.

'Oh, you call Mr Johansen.'

I breathed a sigh of relief. Salvation at last. 'And where's he?'

'Maidstone Hospital,' she replied with a sly grin. 'Twenty-six miles down the road. You can phone him if there's a problem. Is that OK?'

No confidence, no experience, and now no back-up.

'Oh yes, that's just fine,' I said, with as much bitter irony as I could muster. 'As long as there are at least half a dozen patients still living after the weekend, everything will be perfect.'

She pushed some charts across the counter to me with another of those warming smiles.

'You'll be fine,' she said kindly. 'Everybody always is, in the end.'

And then with just a hint of a twinkle in her eye she added carelessly, 'The first six months are the worst. Now, the charts. Could you write up some fluids for these patients for me?'

A sea of odd-looking hieroglyphics met my eyes. I could not make much sense of it.

'Fluids?' I said desperately.

'Yes, fluids.'

I thought quickly. 'What have you got?' I asked, hoping for a clue.

'Oh, all the usual,' she said airily, with a sort of 'Is he really that stupid?' look on her face.

He was. Even now, as an experienced GP, there are times when I look, or feel, completely foolish. At times like that it helps if you have appeared life's most incompetent idiot at a very early stage in your career, so with tremendous foresight, I decided to do just that, right there and then.

'How about some orange juice, then?' I suggested feebly. She stared at me with an incredulous look on her face. 'Lemonade?' The other more junior nurses were gathering round, beginning to get interested in this strange specimen who had just materialised in their midst. 'Ribena? Tea and coffee?' Silence. 'I didn't know you had to write up their drinks.'

One of the junior nurses sniggered, and then snorted loudly. I looked around wildly for a pickaxe to start digging a hole I could fall into, and soon.

The silence returned. As my face grew more like a beetroot with each passing moment, an air of fascination settled upon my ever enlarging audience. I'm sure the patients were all nudging their beds that little bit closer, eager not to miss the entertainment of a lifetime. We all held our breath, waiting, and finally Sister Whitehead proclaimed:

'Drip,' she said, very slowly and deliberately. 'Intravenous. Drip. The clear liquid stuff in those bags,' pointing to a nearby patient who appeared to be in the final stages of apoplexy, 'that runs down those bendy tubey things into the patient's army-warmy to help make them a teeny weeny bit better when they are feeling very, very sick.'

My turn. 'Aha,' I said, stroking my chin seriously. 'You mean *those* sorts of fluids.' I paused for dramatic effect, or something like that. 'What sort of *those* fluids have you got?'

I swear I heard patients running up the stairs from the ward below, curious not to miss out.

She pronounced her verdict, after due consideration. 'Dr

81

Sparrow,' she asked carefully, 'have you ever been on a ward before?'

There was only one way out and I took it. I grovelled.

'Look,' I said, 'can I be blunt?'

'If you can't be the least bit knowledgeable,' she countered, but the twinkle was back in her eye.

'I might as well admit it,' I said. 'I'm hopeless. I know nothing. I've attended very little as a student and I'm sure I only qualified because the typist spelt somebody else's name incorrectly. You can teach me far more than I could ever teach you, and I'll need your help to get through this. But I'll learn quickly, I'll never need telling anything twice and I haven't anywhere near the depth of knowledge to suffer from white coat syndrome . . .'

This, I should explain, is a peculiar arrogance that afflicts newly qualified doctors who see themselves as a superior being the moment they change their student's short white coat for the long one of the doctor. Once acquired, this syndrome stays with you for life. Longer, if you're an orthopaedic surgeon.

'. . . Will you help me out?'

I think I was so pathetic, and so obviously speaking the truth, that they took pity on me. They looked after me wonderfully on that ward from then on, and by the end of six months there was an outside chance that I might one day be almost competent. I owe them a great deal – but they never let me forget my first day and if ever I should show a hint of burgeoning arrogance – we none of us can help it, once in a while – Sister Whitehead would just look at me with a twinkle in her eye and mouth silently, 'Drip.'

As you progress through each house job you begin to learn the wily ways of some of the local GPs.

Most of us, of course, are dedicated, caring, empathic professionals who are only too happy to put ourselves out for the benefit of our patients, even to our own detriment. Our goal is always to look after the sick and the needy in their own homes for as long as we possibly can. We wouldn't dream of shovelling them off to the already overburdened general hospital down the road at the first sign of a cough, or the second bout of diarrhoea, or a temperature of just 0.1 degree above normal.

But then there are the Friday Afternooners . . .

It is Friday afternoon, and your weekend on call.

The next two days stretch enticingly ahead of you. Saturday morning surgery, and then a round of golf, dinner with friends, send the wife and kids off to her mother's – 'Sorry dear, love to come, you know I would, but the patients, they may need me. Do give her my regards,' – and the minute she is out of the door it's feet up, television on, and all the Sunday papers to make your leisurely way through without interruption.

Sheer, unadulterated bliss . . . but at three o'clock there's a call to old Mrs Pengelly.

She lives on her own a few miles out of town, and you visit grudgingly, hoping it is something really simple that will not disturb the vision you have of your weekend to come. She has a temperature, is feeling faint, and has 'come over all funny like' on a couple of occasions, but she is sitting up in bed looking pink and comparatively comfortable.

You ask a few questions, complete your examination, and still have absolutely no idea what is wrong with her. So now you have two options.

You can reassure her, saying that it is early days yet, and promise to visit again tomorrow, and Sunday, and – gritting your teeth – even during the night, if necessary. You can contact her family, neighbours, friends, social services, meals-on-wheels, the district nurse . . . you can do all this, and care for her in the way she so obviously deserves, and is entitled to, and bugger up your entire weekend for good.

Or you can exaggerate all her symptoms, and admit her to hospital. One phone call as against a weekend of hard labour . . . You reach for the phone.

Welcome to the world of the Friday Afternooners.

The trouble with the Friday Afternooners when you are working in a hospital, of course, is that they operate the same admission policy all week long.

As a houseman you spend your days like a cricketer in the nets, constantly fending away as much as you can from all that is thrown at you. Every now and then a GP dispatches a vicious bouncer, and you duck, admit defeat, and reluctantly accept the patient on to the ward.

It is a game we all play – housemen continuously trying to keep them at bay, GPs resorting to all manner of tactics to get them in. But in the end, if the GP really wants the patient to come in, then they do, by one means or another – even if it means that the houseman or casualty officer merely sends them straight back home again.

In this, my first job, I was naïve to the point of stupidity. Ten days into the fray, I was already exhausted beyond anything I had encountered before. I lay fully clothed on the bed in the on-call room at the end of the ward, fast asleep when the telephone rang.

Even at this early stage of my career I had mastered the 'Pick it up before the second ring' reflex, and by the time I was muttering, 'Yeah, it's Dr Sparrow,' I had the light on and was inwardly groaning, having glanced at the cheap bedside clock on the even cheaper bedside table.

2.40 a.m. Oh great.

'It is Dr Kowalski here,' came a voice I would soon learn to dread, 'I have a patient for you. His name is – '

'What's wrong with him?' I interrupted. 'Give me a few details.'

'His name,' persisted Kowalski, 'is Arthur Bidlake, and his address . . .' He ran through the incipient patient's date of birth and marital status and I am sure would have moved on to his inside leg measurement and favourite TV programme had I not interrupted again.

'Yes, but what is actually *wrong* with him?'

I was beginning to get an inkling of the first rule of the game – the more a GP tells you of the patient's details, the less they will tell you about the condition they are trying to admit them with.

'He has a ruptured bladder,' came the dramatic answer. 'He must come into hospital at once, please.'

Now, were this to have happened today I would of course have taken the line 'Interesting diagnosis, Dr Kowalski. What makes you think that, then? Double-decker bus parked on his stomach, perhaps?' But young and befuddled by lack of sleep as I was, I just thought to myself, Ruptured bladder, eh? Sounds sort of serious, followed by, Nifty bit of diagnosis for a GP. This chap must know what he's on about, all right.

'Better send him in, then,' I grunted, rang the ward to confirm his admission, and then fell fast asleep once more.

An hour later, I was standing at the end of the bed containing the newly arrived Arthur Bidlake.

Now, I had never at this stage of my career seen a patient with a ruptured bladder, but I was willing to bet my inaugural month's salary that Arthur Bidlake was not about to be the first of them. He looked just too well, damn him. Old, certainly, grey-haired, dishevelled and not too fussy in the hygiene department, maybe, but basically . . . well!

I stared at him for a moment, and he stared back.

What he was thinking I have not the faintest idea, but my thought processes were crystal clear. Did I actually have to touch this man, or could I persuade one of the nurses to do it for me?

Some nurses really are angels. 'Would you like a bit of help, Mike?' came a soft voice in my ear, and I turned to find I was no longer standing at the end of the bed on my own. Sarah, a young, slightly plump but undeniably pretty staff nurse with short dark hair and just that little something that made you want to get to know her better, was standing there with me.

I nodded thankfully. 'Are you sure?'

She held up her hands in front of me. 'I have gloves,' she said solemnly, 'and a bit of a cold. And you wouldn't know where to start, all on your own, now would you?'

I grinned, and she began painstakingly to undress Arthur. Everything about him was grey, from his matted hair and his complexion to his mud-spattered overcoat, down to the outer of his two aged string vests. I started to ask him some questions while she worked.

'How are you feeling, Mr Bidlake?'

'Quite well, thank you doctor, considering,' he wheezed in reply.

Considering what? I thought to myself. Considering he was supposed to have a ruptured bladder?

'Are you in any pain?' I inquired.

'No, I can't say I'm in any pain,' came the answer. This rather threw me, for a moment.

'Have you been hit by any double-decker buses lately?' I asked, not meaning it to come out loud.

Arthur looked at me with slightly uneasy curiosity, pretending he hadn't understood the question, while Sarah snorted deliciously as she bent over his boots and began to unlace them. 'Been sniffing the nitrous oxide again?' she said, a grin half-hidden on her face.

'No, that comes later,' I said, smiling weakly back. 'Professional joke, sort of. GP sent him in with a suspected ruptured bladder – only know one way he might have managed it.'

By this stage, Sarah had got down to his trousers, and undoing them with expertly concealed distaste she slid them down to his ankles and stood back for a moment, to let me see.

'Well, something's ruptured, all right,' she said flatly, 'but I don't think it's his bladder.'

Staring us in the face, beneath Arthur Bidlake's grey string vest, was Arthur Bidlake's even greyer long johns, grey catheter, and grey catheter bag, leaking perceptibly through a tap that was incompletely turned off. Sarah reached gently forward and gave it a half turn to the left.

'Problem solved,' she said. 'You can take the credit, but it will cost you a drink or two.'

'Three,' I agreed readily. 'Even four, come to think of it. Thank you, Sarah – let's pack him up and get him out of here, shall we?' I turned to walk away to my room again when a thought struck me.

'Mr Bidlake,' I asked curiously, 'tell me. Did Dr Kowalski not examine you when he came round to your house?'

'No,' replied Arthur, giving me a strange look.

'Didn't examine you at all?' I persisted.

'No, didn't come round to the house,' explained Arthur. 'Said he would arrange it all over the telephone for me . . .'

I learned, after that. Take nothing at face value.

Many years later, now gamekeeper turned poacher, I was sitting in the local police station at 3 a.m. with John, a large shambling young man who kept muttering 'Just wanna go back. Let me out and I just wanna go back.'

The police had picked him up in the dark of the night wandering along the central reservation of the motorway, and had brought him into the station for his own protection. I, lucky chap that I was, was the duty police surgeon at the time, and had been called in to undertake a mental health assessment.

This was frequently a long, laborious process involving a psychiatrist, a psychiatric social worker (both of whom would be in entirely different parts of the county, asleep, and reluctant to travel vast distances in the middle of the night) and a recalcitrant patient ranging in condition from the pleasantly nutty to the stark staring fruit-cake variety who believed they were neither ill nor in need of hospitalisation.

But John was different.

'Came out three days ago,' he said mournfully. 'Being treated for depression, I was. They said I was better now, but I'm not, you can see I'm not, can't you?'

I could.

'Kill myself if I have to go on like this any longer. Would have thrown myself under a car, next minute, I would have, but the police car was the first one to come along once I'd made up my mind. Can I just go back, doctor?' he pleaded, raising his eyes to mine. 'I need to go back for more treatment, I know I do.'

'Of course you can, John,' I reassured him, relaxing. Perfect – a single phone call to the hospital and I could be off back to bed within minutes instead of perching on a hard seat in a dimly lit corridor in the police station waiting for the psychiatrist and social worker to drive through the night to a place they wanted to be at even less than I did.

If that were that possible . . .

'Got no beds,' came the disinterested voice over the phone when I eventually got through to the doctor on call.

'What do you mean, got no beds?' I queried, aghast. What the hell was I going to do with him now?

'I mean – got no beds,' repeated the voice. 'You'll have to try somewhere else,' and the line clicked dead just as I screeched back at him 'What do you mean, try somewhere else? There isn't anywhere else.'

I hadn't even got as far as mentioning John's name, let alone his pressing need for admission.

I put the phone down and sat thinking for a moment. A psychiatric hospital without any beds . . . And then I went and spoke to John again, and asked him some different questions. After all, he had only left there three days earlier . . .

I rang the hospital again and asked to be put through to the emergency male ward.

'Hi, it's Dr Sparrow here,' I said breezily. 'I had just arranged admission for my patient, John Burbin, when I was cut off from the SHO. Just checking you have a free bed for him.'

'Of course we do,' came back the friendly male voice. 'John not well again? Of course we'll take him back.'

And then I rang the doctor again.

'Dr Sparrow here,' I said icily. 'Just to let you know that John Burbin is en route to one of those beds you said you didn't have, and that my report on the matter will be with your consultant, the GMC and the local papers by midday tomorrow. Do have a nice day, won't you?' and then I replaced the receiver with intricate care.

It helps, in the end, if you know how to play the game just that little bit better than they do.

So you get used to the local GPs in the course of a hospital job.

Like Dr Ashwood – Anna – who frequently rang for advice, but rarely actually sent a patient in.

'Hi, it's Anna Ashwood here,' she would say breathily. 'I think I might have an early appendicitis here, and I'd welcome your advice.'

'How long have they had the pain?' I soon learned to ask.

'Oh, an hour or so. It's on the left at the moment, and not too bad, but it could move to the right, couldn't it, later in the day and get worse and I might have to wake you up in the night and – '

'I'm prepared to take that risk,' I announced solemnly, 'if you are. Have you considered waiting a while to see what happens?'

'Oh thanks, *thanks* for your help,' she would gush. 'I do *so* appreciate it.'

Or Dr Endacott, a forbidding grey-haired man in his late fifties who had formerly been a surgeon.

'Endacott here,' he would announce in clipped tones. 'Renal colic for you – given him pethidine, Stemetil and atropine – may need some more before you arrange his emergency IVP' (a special contrast X-ray looking for kidney stones). 'And don't forget to check his calcium levels, will you . . . ?'

But for the King of the Friday Afternooners you could not top Dr Ian Benjamin.

It began slowly, insidiously.

A patient of his, admitted via casualty with a suspected heart attack ended up on my surgical ward after a quick detour via intensive care. By the time he got to me, four people (plus or minus Dr Benjamin – I was never quite certain whether he had actually seen the patient or not) had diagnosed him as having gall-stones, and who was I to disagree?

I perched on the end of his bed and began checking his medication on admission, as no doubt others had prior to me. He had quite an impressive list, so I carefully ran through them one by one, noting the reason for each until I came to the last.

'Zantac,' I read out to him. 'Did they start you on that when you came in here?'

'No,' said the patient, a rather tired and faded man in his late fifties. 'Dr Benjamin put me on it some time ago for my heart.'

'Not for your heart,' I said, shaking my head. 'It reduces the amount of acid your stomach produces – it's for ulcers, indigestion and so forth.'

'Don't have nothing wrong with my stomach,' he persisted.

He was probably just a bit confused, I thought, but I was curious. For once the ward was quiet, and I looked up Dr Benjamin's number and gave the surgery a ring.

'I'm sorry, but the surgery is now closed for the day,' said a well-bred lady's voice on the answering machine. 'If you have a problem that may not keep until tomorrow morning, please go to the casualty department at St Benedict's, where they will be pleased to attend to you.'

Oh, will they indeed? I thought to myself.

I rang again the next day, receiving the same message, and again the day after. And then the daily rigours of being a junior houseman took over once more, and I forgot all about it.

Two weeks later another of Dr Benjamin's patients arrived on the ward, again via casualty, with a case of haemorrhoids to be proud of. The poor chap was in agony.

Having clerked him in and decided upon his treatment, I scanned the list of drugs he was on.

'Do you get indigestion?' I asked.

'No, never,' he grimaced. 'Jesus, doc, can you give me something for the pain? Bloody killing me, these piles are.'

'Yes, it's on the way,' I nodded. 'Nice big needle and an ice pack. I . . . um . . . see you're taking Zantac. Can you tell me why?'

'Touch of bronchitis,' he said, tapping his chest. 'Too many cigarettes.'

I nodded again. 'I see,' I said as if it was of no consequence, and walked back to the nurses' station, deep in thought.

This time I got through to the surgery at the first attempt. The same mellifluous well-bred voice, but this time in person, not on a machine.

'May I speak to Dr Benjamin, please?'

'I'm sorry,' came the meticulously polite reply, 'but I'm afraid he is not in this morning. Would you like to try again this afternoon?'

I did like, but lo and behold: 'I'm sorry, but the surgery is now closed for the day . . .'

So when was the bloody place open? I wondered.

'Between nine and eleven each morning,' came the well-modulated reply the following day, with just a hint of frost in the voice.

'And afternoons?'

'Dr Benjamin is not always in in the afternoons. You will have to ring and check his availability.'

'That's . . .' the line went dead, '. . . just what I thought I was doing,' I finished to myself. Did this guy actually work for a living?

At dinner in the doctors' mess that evening I sat next to Andrew, the house physician on the opposite wards to myself. A big amiable brute of a rugby player, he was more at home with a fire extinguisher in his hands after a few beers than a stethoscope on the wards – 'At least I know how to use a fire extinguisher properly,' he would admit with a sheepish grin.

He treated house jobs like a fifteen-a-side game – put your head down at the start and keep charging towards the other end until somebody blows a whistle and you can stop, the torture at last over.

'Come across a GP called Benjamin?' I asked mildly.

'Pah,' he snorted, shovelling a mountainous helping of steak and kidney pie into the yawning gap between nose and chin, 'come across his patients, more like, mostly in casualty. They seem to think he's wonderful, whenever they can get to see him – always so busy, they say, which I interpret as being "Never there when you want him." Always trying them on the latest and best drugs, no complaint too minor to treat. Rattle like pill boxes when they come in, most of them.'

'Any of his on the ward at the moment?'

'A few – two came in this morning. Usual load of rubbish. "Tired for a day." "Been coughing all morning" – that sort of thing.'

'Mind if I take a look?'

He halted, heavily laden fork suspended in front of his wide-open mouth, and gave me a disbelieving stare.

'Be my guest. Not enough work of your own to do?'

'Oh, just curious. Passes the time, you know.'

'Yeah, right,' said Andrew sardonically, before turning his attention back to the weightier matters in hand and losing interest completely.

I saw Andrew's patients later that evening, and found some interesting drug combinations on their prescription sheets. In all of them, at the bottom, was the aforementioned Zantac. One patient had indigestion and claimed that Zantac was unhelpful, but that Benjamin had insisted he continue it. 'Six months I've been on it,' he said. 'No use as yet, but if my doctor says to keep trying . . .'

Another thought he might be on it for his kidneys, and a third maybe for arthritis. The last one muttered something about his ingrowing toenails, but then he did have a very high temperature at the time . . .

And there the matter might have ended, idle curiosity on a junior doctor's part. You have to remember that I was a young, inexperienced house surgeon, and Dr Benjamin a highly respected – if rarely available – GP of some standing in the community, who no doubt had forgotten much that I had as yet to get around to learning. Who was I to question what he did?

But three weeks later fate took a hand.

Andrew and I had made a foray into town on one of the few evenings we had off together, and were heading for any pub that might have some beer in it, followed by any party that might let us in.

'Hey,' said Andrew suddenly, holding an arm in front of my chest. He pointed in the direction of a short, stout, dark-haired man climbing out of a shiny new Daimler. 'That's your Dr Benjamin.'

'So how on earth does he manage to afford one of those?' I wondered, 'and on a couple of hours' work a day, if you're lucky. Whatever he's got, I'd like some of it.'

There was something about Benjamin's behaviour that caught the eye, and we stood and watched for a moment. There was a certain shiftiness about his movements: he looked round furtively before scurrying across the road and disappearing behind a terrace of shops.

'What's he up to, then?' mused Andrew. 'Shall we take a little look?'

We followed him discreetly, or as discreetly as two junior doctors are able to do anything, and as we turned the corner at the back of the end shop, a bakery, we could see Benjamin look carefully around him before giving a staccato tap on a door hidden in the shadows. A beam of light suddenly erupted into the darkness, and then Benjamin was gone, swallowed up in the recess of whatever lay beyond.

'One, two, three, four,' counted Andrew. 'Fourth shop along. Come on, let's take a look.'

We made our way back round to the frontage again, past the baker's, the grocer's and the newsagent's, and came to rest in front of the darkened facade of the fourth.

'So that's what he's up to,' murmured Andrew, showing a quicker speed of thought than either of us would have previously given him credit for. 'The devious old so and so . . .'

Back in the early eighties, two drugs were launched in quick succession that revolutionised the treatment of peptic (caused by acid) ulcers. Then, as now, each drug had two names – firstly the generic name, which was the name of the actual compound, and secondly the trade name. This was the brand name given to the drug for marketing purposes by the company that made it – usually something catchy and simple so that we poor doctors could remember it.

Ranitidine (brand name Zantac) and cimetidine (brand name Tagamet) were, and still are, excellent drugs. They were soon widely used, dramatically reducing the number of perforated ulcers we saw as acute surgical admissions almost overnight – not to mention the number of deaths resulting from what was a serious condition.

But they came at a price – namely around £30 per month for Zantac, which at the time was highly expensive.

The world of prescribing works as follows. Dispensing doctors and chemists have to buy in all the drugs they dispense in advance and are reimbursed each time they fulfil a prescription, at a set price for each drug. This would usually be the manufacturer's cost price plus around ten per cent.

So if you bought Zantac from the company that made it at say £30 a box, and were reimbursed £33 each time you prescribed it, you made £3 profit, which is how chemists make a living and dispensing doctors pay their mortgage.

But just supposing . . .

We were standing in front of a high street chemist.

'You know Ali, my registrar,' said Andrew. 'He was telling me one day how they produce all these drugs illegally in India, Pakistan, Thailand . . . all over the place. Britain won't allow them to be used here because they flout the patent laws, and the quality is suspect in any case, but they do have one thumping great advantage.'

'Which is?' I asked, my mind racing ahead.

'They're dirt cheap. Zantac is £1, maybe £2 a box. Imagine if you could get them for that price, ship them over here and prescribe them for £33 a go. Say £30 profit, per patient, per month. A hundred patients . . .' He did a quick mental calculation. '. . . around £36,000 per year. Two hundred patients . . . £72,000. Say his practice has, what, three or four thousand patients? How many could he prescribe Zantac to without anybody beginning to notice? Three hundred? Four hundred?'

I was beginning to follow his train of thought.

'Look at what he's using it for,' continued Andrew excitedly. 'Coughs, kidney problems. Suppose he was using it on five hundred patients, maybe. That would net him getting on for two hundred grand a year on just the one drug alone, and look at all the other drugs his patients come into hospital on. He's probably got an entire fleet of Daimlers parked in a mansion somewhere . . .'

Which is exactly how it turned out. Benjamin had a profit-sharing agreement with the chemist, who just happened to be his brother-in-law, and his brother-in-law had a relative who just happened to be a shipping agent somewhere in Asia . . . and so it went on.

I have no idea how many doctors and chemists the scheme ultimately involved, because Andrew and I had long moved on before the investigation was completed, and I equally have no idea what became of all those involved in the long term.

But in the short term . . .

We moved on from our deliberations to a pub, and then another, and to an exuberant party followed by another even more exuberant than the first. The last I saw of Andrew that evening he was staggering around in his element with – yes, you've guessed it – a fire extinguisher in his hands shouting at the top of his voice 'Anyone think they're on fire here? Let me come and put you out.'

I left him to it.

The next day, being a Sunday, was another day off for the pair of us. I slept late, rising shortly before lunch, and wandered down to Andrew's room to see if he had surfaced. A strange groaning sound could be heard from within.

Andrew was sitting on the side of his bed holding his head in his hands as if it was in danger of falling off any second. 'Never again,' he muttered feebly, 'don't let me do it ever again.'

Something caught my eye by the foot of the bed, and I picked it up, grinning.

'So where did you let off the fire extinguisher, Andrew?' I asked in the tone of a father gently chastising an errant son.

Another groan, followed by an 'Oh, my God,' and then 'I walked home,' he told me bit by bit, piecing the memories together, 'and just as I was passing that chemist's again I saw Benjamin's car pulling away, and got curious. So I went round the back and there were two other blokes there, just finishing unloading a lorry – big round containers, I saw one of them.'

I could imagine the scene.

'Then the lorry drove off, and I thought I would go over to the door and take a look inside . . .'

'They'd left it unlocked for you, then, had they?' I asked facetiously. 'That was nice of them.'

'Not . . . actually unlocked, no,' said Andrew slowly, 'but sort of . . . a bit loose, if you know what I mean, so I gave it a gentle nudge . . .'

'The sort of gentle nudge that you get from a ten or fifteen yard run-up?'

'Yes,' he nodded, wishing immediately that he hadn't, 'that sort of gentle nudge. Inside there were some steps down to a store room, and inside that a whole shit load of containers of imported drugs. When I took the tops off them the tablets were all loose, not foil-packed or anything, and I thought about Benjamin and his Daimler and how bloody hard we both work for peanuts and how he'd probably get away with it all and I was wondering what we should do about it when I remembered something else.'

'Which was?'

'When one of Benjamin's patients was on the ward he showed me these Zantac he was taking, and I thought they didn't look quite right and perhaps he had just put some other tablets in the wrong bottle. You know how incredibly stupid some patients can be. So I chucked them in the sink in the sluice room, and . . . pass me a glass of water, there's a good chap, before I die of thirst.'

'And?' I pressed him. 'What did you do, Andrew?'

'. . . and I let off the fire extinguisher and blasted the whole ruddy lot of them,' he said, a huge grin spreading across his face at the memory. 'These foreign tablets, they're not the same as the proper ones made over here.'

'Let me guess,' I said, beginning to laugh.

'Yes,' he said, his shoulders starting to shake. 'They're dissolvable.'

6

A Hint of Violence

The world of medicine after you qualify – especially in general practice – is essentially devoid of violent confrontation. I appreciate it can be very different for inner city GPs with bars on their windows, panic buttons in their surgeries and an ever recurring nightmare on the streets during house calls, particularly at night, but in rural practice life is generally calm and trouble-free.

Many years ago, however, I was doing a spell as a locum in a town in the Midlands for a GP who was temporarily indisposed. It was the early hours of the morning, and I was returning to my car after visiting a young lad with appendicitis. As I rounded the corner I could see three youths sitting nonchalantly on the bonnet of my car, who seemed disinclined to move – until I threw myself into the driving seat, started the engine, and they realised with alarm that the car was moving itself, in reverse, and at some speed.

In those days I always made sure that I undertook night-time visits looking as little like a doctor as possible – which, to be honest, at that stage in my career required the minimum of disguise – and travelled normally in jeans, denim jacket and trainers. Under no circumstance would you find me with a stethoscope draped carelessly round my neck, or carrying the traditional black bag. You might as well have paraded down the street with a sandwich board announcing, 'Hey, boys, I'm a doctor. Come along and mug me right now.'

My equipment would be in a rucksack, occasionally even a supermarket carrier bag, and I was then young enough, fit enough and confident enough to think I could deal adequately with any situation that might arise. Many doctors were justifiably nervous of night calls, and how some of the female GPs managed to cope with the worst of the places they had to visit is beyond me.

Life as a student had prepared me well for some of these encounters. Before you qualify pretty much anything goes, and frequently does. I can vaguely recall nearly losing my life when encountering the entire Australian rugby team in a bar close to Bayswater and engaging in a somewhat fraught conversation with a six foot seven inch second row forward. 'Do you think you're really big enough to play rugby?' I asked curiously.

Steam began to emanate from his nostrils, but it wasn't until I ventured to ask if his mother still washed behind his ears that it seemed somehow more than he could cope with.

Some people may have learned the art of self-defence by mis-spending their youth in a boxing ring, but at Mary's it was all part of the student curriculum – or at least, the unofficial one. By which I mean the pre-match skirmishes of 'The Hospitals Rugby Cup' – a vicious battle on the pitch between rival rugby teams, preceded by several weeks of even more vicious battles off the pitch between rival sets of supporters.

Hostilities would range from dumping the odd abandoned car on the opponent's home territory, wheels removed and daubed with less than complimentary slogans, to a full blown raid on the opposition's medical school. On one occasion we cemented a complete toilet to the steps outside the front of the London Hospital Medical School entrance, preventing them from being able to open the main door. Another found us in St Bartholomew's Medical School bar, attempting to steal their prized mascot, surrounded by an angry contingent of home fans with only our crowbars and pickaxes with which to defend ourselves . . .

All good clean fun, I promise you, and no actual fatalities.

The first potentially violent confrontation I came across was as a junior surgeon, four months into my first job. By this stage I had learned a few lessons of survival – like, if you think a patient may turn out to have violent tendencies, try and get him admitted on to somebody else's ward in the first place.

Elderly people often become confused when admitted to hospital, particularly at night. A change of circumstances, feeling unwell, a loss of all the stabilising influences of their home environment . . . anything might happen, and frequently does.

'Need you in the ward,' came the urgent voice of the ward sister over the phone one evening. 'Got a possible jumper in bed number one.'

'A jumper,' I repeated slowly. 'As in "pullover", or as in "throwing oneself off the top of a high building"?'

'Just get here, Mike, if you would,' she said exasperatedly, 'preferably before I only need you to confirm his death.'

The ward was in a state of turmoil.

All the available staff were gathered around the foot of the first bed as you entered, which should have contained one Edward James Baker, but currently was merely supporting his right foot. This rested precariously on the iron bed-head, whilst his left was planted more firmly on the windowsill next to a large window which was wide open, and through which a hefty draught was entering.

The good Mr Baker was no doubt a little on the cold side, having apparently neglected to put on his pyjamas. He stood there, stark naked, shouting furiously, with a clear bottle grasped firmly in both hands, raised in a threatening manner.

'Come any closer and I'll jump,' he bellowed. 'Leave me alone, damn you, damn all of you. Nobody cares about me, nobody . . .'

The man in the next bed was an unpleasant individual recovering from a hernia operation. He was greatly put out because he had demanded a private room on admission only to be told none was available.

'Disgraceful behaviour,' he said shrilly. 'Don't see why I should have to put up with this. I'll be writing to my MP as soon as I'm out of here. Disgraceful, indeed. You . . .' pointing at me as I arrived amongst the happy band of onlookers, '. . . you're the doctor. Why don't you do something useful?'

'OK,' I said cheerfully. 'Shut up, and stop making the situation any worse than it already is. There, will that do you?'

He opened his mouth, spluttering, and then closed it again, catching the thunderous look on my face. 'Later,' you could almost hear his brain whirring, 'I'll be writing to my MP about you, too.'

I stood for a moment, completely nonplussed. They didn't teach us about moments like this, in medical school.

Mr Baker had been admitted for assessment of an as yet undiagnosed abdominal mass, and had been quiet, almost withdrawn, for the past couple of days. What had triggered this sudden change of character I had absolutely no idea, and for the moment it was unimportant. Something had to be done, and soon.

'I suppose,' I whispered to the ward sister standing next to me, 'you've already tried the "Now be a good chap, Mr Baker, and come on down this instant before you make a bloody mess in the car park" approach?'

'Only for the last half an hour,' she hissed back. 'I even shouted at him to stop behaving as badly as that bloke in the next bed, and you can see how successful that was, can't you? Like – not very successful at all.'

'Then why don't we just rush him?' I suggested. 'We should hopefully be able to grab him before he's had a chance to throw himself out.'

'And we might not,' came the sensible reply. 'Besides, just take another look at that bottle he has so carefully cradled in his hands. Firstly, it's made of glass, and secondly, have you noticed exactly what's in it? You can rush him if you like, but nobody else is going to have a go at it.'

I took a second look, as suggested, and let out an involuntary

'Aaah.' In Mr Baker's clutches . . . was Mr Baker's urine bottle, and Mr Baker's urine bottle was full to the point of overflowing.

'So what on earth are you going to do, Mike?' she urged. 'I really think he's going to jump in a minute.'

'What floor are we on?' I asked, contemplating.

'Third.'

I considered the options. We could send a raiding party to one of the ground-floor wards for all the mattresses they could muster and spread them out below to cushion his fall before he splattered himself on the concrete, but that would take time, and time was one thing that seemed to be in short supply at the moment.

Three floors up . . . and only four feet to the floor. I began to see a way out.

Mr Baker shifted his weight slightly, preparatory to a final lunge wholly on to the sill, and I made my move, almost without thinking, muttering a silent prayer as I did so. 'Whatever happens next, please don't let the urine land all over me.'

I bent down, grabbed hold of the foot of the bed, and tugged it as hard as I could away from the window. Struggling to keep his balance, Mr Baker threw his arms up in the air, relinquishing his hold on the bottle, and toppled over backwards, landing flat on his back on the bed with a thud that knocked all the air out of him.

And the urine bottle, in slow, slow motion, flew up to the ceiling, executed a perfect somersault, and came down fairly and squarely on the chest of the man in the next bed.

I have since then been present on two further occasions when physical force has been used in the world of medicine, both times, I have to say, to great effect. I am just sorry to have to tell you that I was the perpetrator in each case.

In my early career I carried with me the cavalier attitudes of student days into my chosen profession. Nearly twenty years later some might say I do so still.

But the student becomes the doctor and takes with him all that he has learned.

My early sojourn in the North as a junior house physician was a busy but generally untroubled time. Although it pales into insignificance by comparison with today's climate, we did have a problem with the burgeoning local drug culture, and with one individual in particular.

Jason was a heroin addict. This would not normally present me with a problem – we use heroin (diamorphine, to give it its medical name) to help with pain relief, often following heart attacks, whereas some people use it purely to make themselves feel better, but in their case it is illegally. Many doctors have ambivalent feelings towards drug abuse itself, but not towards the problems that come with it.

Invariably in the early hours of the morning Jason would arrive in casualty saying he had taken an overdose, or was in the acute stages of withdrawal and in dire need of medication. When I watch such programmes as *Casualty* on television, I am always struck by the unlimited numbers of dedicated staff available to support, encourage, console and empathise – with other members of the staff, of course, not with the poor old patients. They generally have far less need of such attention.

In the early eighties, however, casualty departments were often barren, desolate areas in the small dark hours where junior doctors were frequently isolated with unpredictable patients.

Caught in the era between *Dixon of Dock Green* and carrying your own CS gas and electrical immobiliser, we struggled along as best we could. In the hospital where I was then working we had a high proportion of female staff, and Jason had an unerring instinct for when they were alone on duty. I sometimes wondered if he actually drew up the hospital rota and handed it in to the chief administrator for distribution.

After several months of his sinister games with the now frankly scared staff, they eventually approached the consultants for some help and guidance. But they neglected to reflect on the realities of life. Consultants were in bed asleep at two o'clock in the morning, sometimes even their own, and junior doctors just had to learn to take the rough with the even rougher as best they could.

I knew all about Jason but we had never met, and probably never would have done had I not been inadvertently invited to the inauguration of the local mayor. A patient left the invitation in casualty one day, and Tippex is such a wonderful invention when used judiciously.

Granted, nobody present had the faintest idea who I was or what I was doing there, and truth to tell, by the end of a splendidly alcoholic evening – especially splendid as it was at somebody else's expense – I was not entirely sure, either.

I was aware, however, as I staggered back to my humble hospital flat (two rooms, one of them even with windows) that the quickest way home was through the casualty department. In addition, I knew they would have black coffee, and lots of it.

And that is how I met Jason, or more precisely how he met me.

He was in casualty, plying his usual trade, as I wandered in. In those days a doctor wearing a suit meant that he was important, and the only important doctors anyone knew of were the consultants. For once I was immaculately be-suited, which by definition made me a consultant – a very young, inebriated and distinctly under-qualified consultant, but a consultant none the less.

I decided to consult him.

Jason was in the process of explaining how much pain he was in, and how he was sure he was going to die. I have to gloss over the details of the next half-hour, even though I doubt whether a criminal prosecution is likely so long after the events of that evening.

I explained to Jason that he wasn't in quite as much pain as he could be, and that the next time he came in he might very well be correct – I would instruct my staff to let him die, as he had so often said he would. We would all of course be completely inconsolable, but we would be alive and inconsolable and some-how I thought that might help.

Strangely – as I was to be reminded the following morning – this conversation appeared not to have taken place in the casualty department itself, but in a dark corner outside the hospital, round the back of the selfsame mortuary where I was suggesting Jason might find himself on his next visit.

The only other feeling permeating my befuddled brain at this stage was the pain in the knuckles of my right hand. I had a pre-monition of the uncanny sensation which has surfaced once or twice more in my subsequent career. It is the one you experience just moments after the General Medical Council have regretfully informed you that you can no longer be a doctor – ever – because Hippocrates never mentioned in his oath that assaulting the patient was all part of the caring process.

What I did was of course unethical, unjustifiable and another un- of some importance – unlawful, that's the word I was looking for. But he never came back, and the casualty department had had a long-standing millstone finally removed from their neck. There was just one small problem left to deal with.

I had to buy a new suit.

The second occasion violence reared its ugly head I have to say I recall with considerable pleasure. I was a house surgeon during the time of the Iraq/Iran war, or one of them. At this stage of my career I was geographically challenged, and could not have begun to tell you where either country was.

I did know, however, that my fellow house officer came from Iran, and the senior registrar from Iraq. Or was it the other way round? It is of course not in the least relevant to this tale that the senior registrar was fat, greasy, odorous, unpleasant and male, and the house officer, Martha, petite, fragrant and devastatingly pretty.

Most physically unattractive men in positions of comparative power in the world of medicine just adore to have pretty junior female staff, and he was no exception. In these enlightened times I am sure that much of what went on then would be obliterated by crew-cut feminists shouting slogans and waving placards – something benign like 'All surgeons are fat chauvinistic pigs.' On this occasion they would have been right.

The registrar, Mr Abraham, used to alternately leer at and then castigate Martha mercilessly, and occasionally contrive to do both at the same time. Generally speaking he would not do this in the presence of other male staff, but would chide her obsequiously and be nauseatingly encouraging. This hideous spectacle was responsible for the only time I was physically sick on the ward when alcohol was not a major contributory factor.

Our already uneasy relationship had all but reached crisis point two weeks earlier.

I had been called down to casualty to see a young eight-year-old lad who had been brought in for assessment after being knocked down by a car. His observations were all fine, and the casualty officer was just about to discharge him when he suddenly winced and started to complain of abdominal pain.

Alarm bells began to ring.

By the time I reached casualty he was in severe discomfort, the colour draining from his face by the second.

'Thinking what I'm thinking?' I asked Helen, the casualty officer, as we stood and looked at the lad.

She nodded. 'Possible ruptured spleen,' she said quietly, trying not to worry the already highly anxious parents who were standing just a few yards to our left.

'Seen one before?' She shook her head. 'Nor have I,' I admitted, 'but . . .'

The 'but' hung in the air between us. A ruptured spleen is a surgical emergency, and if we were correct, this young lad needed to be in theatre, and fast.

Abraham, I knew, was up in his on-call room next to the doctors' mess. I had seen him there with his wife and young child when the call from casualty had first come through. I dialled his room direct.

'Got an eight-year-old down here in casualty with a suspected ruptured spleen,' I said tersely, 'and he's not at all well. Could you come right down?' There was a grunt at the other end of the phone, and the line clicked dead.

Five minutes passed, and there was no sign of him. Helen and I had been busy – Ian, the boy, who was looking progressively greyer by the minute, had had an intravenous drip inserted in his arm, a pre-op medication had been given, and we had spoken to his parents and advised them of the potentially serious nature of his condition.

Trembling, his father had signed the consent form for the operation, technically referred to as a 'laparotomy and proceed' – or in layman's terms, open up his abdomen as wide as you can and get on and deal with whatever it was you found in there.

Still there was no Abraham. I called him again.

'This is getting serious,' I said pointedly. 'I've been here long enough for you to know that I would never ask you to come straight away unless I was really worried. I need you here now,' and I put the phone down myself before he subjected me to another of his grunts.

It was not perhaps the normal way for a junior houseman to address his senior registrar, but these were not normal times. I rang the operating theatre and booked an urgent slot, and contacted the on-call anaesthetist, who couldn't have been more responsive.

'I'll go down to pre-op right away,' he said. 'Anything else I should know?'

'Yes, Abraham hasn't seen him yet,' I admitted. 'This is Helen's and my diagnosis alone, up till now.'

'Good enough for me,' he said. 'Where is the fat tub of lard, anyway?'

There was an unmistakable grunt a few yards behind me. 'The fat tub of lard has just slithered into casualty,' I replied quietly.

'See you in a moment,' and there was a chuckle at the other end of the phone.

Abraham had moved through into the cubicle where Ian was lying, now semi-conscious, his mother sitting by his side, holding his hand and looking terrified. Without so much as a glance in her direction he pulled back the blanket covering Ian and laid a hand heavily on his stomach. Ian cried out in pain.

I took a certain amount of grim satisfaction from the look on Abraham's face as he struggled to admit that Helen and I were right, at which point even he had to admit defeat.

'Better get on and book theatre,' he said grudgingly. 'And get a consent form signed.'

'Already done,' I said icily.

'Then contact the on-call anaesthetist.'

'I have. He's ready and waiting. It's you we've been hanging on for.'

Abraham grunted again, and turned to walk away.

'Doctor,' called Ian's mother to his retreating back, 'my son – is he going to be all right?'

He half turned to face her. 'Now that I'm here,' he said, and walked off down the corridor in the direction of the operating theatre.

'And thank you for that vote of confidence, Mr Abraham,' murmured Helen in my ear, re-entering the cubicle. 'Nice company you keep, Mike. Anything I can do?'

'Mmm. You hold him down and I'll hit him. Got any porters?'

'Good lord no – this is a hospital casualty department. What on earth would make you think we'd have any hospital porters available in an emergency?'

Several years previously, when I was a student, there was a strike involving one of the hospital unions, and I literally bumped into Sir Graham Parker, then the Queen's gynaecologist, negotiating (rather badly) a trolley from the corridor into the lift. On the trolley lay a semi-conscious patient.

'Ah, young Sparrow,' he said, registering my surprise. 'Thought I was too proud to push a trolley, maybe?'

'Um . . .' I spluttered, having probably thought exactly that.

'Patient needs an operation, I need them in theatre,' he continued, smiling benignly. 'Like to give me a hand with the other end?'

So if it was good enough for Sir Graham . . .

'OK then, Helen. Would you like to take the head or the feet?'

We wheeled Ian at speed down the long corridor, spun round a corner and surged through the swing doors into theatre reception.

'One ruptured spleen reporting for duty,' I said. 'I'm off to get scrubbed up. Helen, you wouldn't have another quick word with Ian's mum and dad for me, would you? Sort of forgot them in the rush.'

'Of course,' she said, 'but it will cost you later,' and she strolled off back into the corridor, where Ian's parents were waiting.

I changed into the surgical greens and walked through to the washroom to scrub up.

'Abraham already inside?' I asked the theatre sister, who was just being assisted into her sterilised gown.

'Haven't seen him,' she said, surprised. 'I presumed he would be coming in with you. Wherever he is, he'd better get here soon. Poor kid looks awful.'

My heart sank. Where on earth had he got to?

'See the organ grinder's here,' said the anaesthetist, patting me on the shoulder as he entered the room. 'No sign of the monkey?'

'I assumed he had come straight here from casualty,' I said grimly. 'Looks like I assumed wrong.'

I stopped washing and dashed out of the theatre, raced up to the doctors' mess and burst into Abraham's room without bothering to knock. No sign of him anywhere, or his family. I sped back out into the corridor, clattering down the stairs, looking this way and that, and then at last I caught sight of him, leading his wife and daughter out through the main door. What the hell did the man think he was doing?

One last charge down the corridor and I was out through the front door behind them, into the car park and across to where by this time he was helping his wife into the car.

'We're ready for you,' I gasped. 'Are you coming, or what?'

He looked disparagingly at me through his piggy little eyes. 'I'm just taking my wife home,' he said menacingly.

'You're what?' I exploded. 'I've got an eight- year-old kid bleeding to death in theatre and you're taking your wife home?' I knew he lived a good twenty minutes away from the hospital. 'You want me to contact the duty undertaker now, or should I just go and find another surgeon to take over instead?'

I think it was 'another surgeon' that did it. I really think he was stubborn enough and stupid enough to take his family home, knowing that our consultant – both his and my boss – was off sick for a few days, and there was no way he would have wanted to lose face in front of his wife to an angry young junior surgeon standing in lime green surgical pyjamas in the hospital car park before a rapidly gathering crowd of interested onlookers, but 'another surgeon' . . .

He operated, and Ian, who did indeed have a ruptured spleen, survived. But another forty minutes or more . . . who knows what might have happened.

'Houseman 1, Registrar 0,' murmured the anaesthetist, clapping me on the shoulder again as we stood talking in the changing rooms when it was all over. 'But watch your back, there's a good chap. You still have to work with the man.'

And here was that man now.

We were part way through the Friday morning ward round. Abraham was giving Martha a torrid time, enjoying himself hugely into the bargain.

It was not something he would normally do in my presence,

but on this occasion he had obviously decided that although I was present in body I was entirely absent in spirit. This was an assessment I would be forced to agree with in the vast majority of cases, but for once I had arrived on the ward without a hangover. This wasn't my fault, I hasten to point out, as after two nights on call I had fallen asleep in my chair before the pubs had opened.

And what is more, I was even listening to what he was saying, in a sort of dumbstruck horror.

I can no longer recall a single word or phrase, just the impression it formed on me. More importantly, I was acutely aware of the obvious unease and distress of Martha, who was desperately holding back the tears. Even had I had the benefit of a white charger I would no doubt have been entirely incapable of saddling it, yet alone riding in to the rescue, but there was a limit to how much of his foul-mouthed abuse any junior doctor could withstand.

So I told him gently, quietly and I like to think rather diplomatically, 'For God's sake, you fat bastard, leave her alone. You were not, as you seem to think, put upon this earth for the pleasure of the female sex, but merely to make warts look comparatively attractive and promote the longevity of the dung beetle population. Enough excrement in one package to keep an entire dynasty alive. Now either treat her like the lady she is or . . .'

Rather elegantly phrased, don't you think?

At this point I became aware that the entire ward was sitting up in their beds listening avidly to every word I spoke, even the chap in the corner on the life support machine. The only emotion I could detect behind the sneer on Abraham's face was surprise – in part, I believe, because I had strung three and a half sentences together, but mostly due to the fact that obviously no one as insignificant as myself had ever spoken to him in such a manner before. He duly turned his attentions to me, beginning to jab me in the chest with his plump sweaty forefinger.

'Now you listen to me, boy,' he said in what I think he felt was his most domineering tone of voice. 'Your career in medicine hangs in the balance . . .' (of course he was completely wrong, my career had ceased to hang anywhere and fallen off every perch it had ever encountered a long time previously) '. . . and I can make or break you with a flick of my fingers. When I want your opinion, I'll ask for it.'

He continued to jab at a marginally slower rate and I continued to become seriously angry. It is fair to say that many of the strategically important moments of my career have revolved around me looking completely stupid, not to mention ignorant and incompetent, and therefore I think I can allow myself this particular moment of sheer unadulterated bragging.

It was the only time in my fluctuating professional life when I fully understood the meaning of the phrase 'Ice ran through my veins,' which it did, and damn great chunks of the stuff too. For once I knew everyone was awaiting my next move, and uncharacteristically I was beginning to enjoy the limelight.

I looked him squarely in the eye, and said very slowly and calmly, 'If you don't remove your finger from my chest this very second, several people here are going to be required to remove your body from this floor.' Even I was impressed.

The ward held its breath – all apart from the guy on the life support machine, that is, who was busy trying to turn it off so that he could hear a little better. I think that anyone less self-important might have thought twice, but this man merely jabbed again.

So I hit him. As my fist approached his jaw, I was already acknowledging the likely end of my not as yet burgeoning career. As jaw and fist combined, I was getting quite used to the idea, and as his poleaxed body crashed to the floor – well, quite frankly, I no longer cared. It was just one of those great moments in medicine, and perhaps the first of my contributions to a ward round I could be justifiably proud of.

For three or four seconds absolute silence reigned. This was the 'Did he really do that?' interlude, and then suddenly all the patients and staff started clapping and cheering. Years of studying the 1966 World Cup Final stood me in good stead.

I raised my arms in the air in my best Geoff Hurst salute, turned, and strolled calmly off the ward, the applause ringing in my ears.

I was almost half-way down the stairs before it occurred to me that I had just knocked out the man who was due to perform an emergency laparotomy in theatre in twenty minutes' time . . .

7

More Tales from the Wards

Several months into my second job after qualification I was beginning to feel passably confident. This is the dangerous illusion of competence you develop when you have yet to kill a patient, and I had survived nine months' labour without so doing.

This is by no means so flippant as it sounds. The majority of doctors, sooner or later, will kill a patient by making a mistake. In my first job there was a surgeon that I respected – a rare breed, to be sure, but they do exist – who took me aside with some serious advice. At this stage of my career I wanted greatly to become a surgeon myself, so for once I listened to what he had to say.

'If you only remember one thing, Mike, remember this,' he said cryptically. 'You will never become a good surgeon, or even a good doctor, until you have filled an entire graveyard with your mistakes.'

Our village graveyard remains half empty, despite my best endeavours as a GP over the past ten years. Does that mean that I have a long way to go before I succeed in becoming a good GP, or that I have exceeded my expectations and kept my patients alive longer than anyone could possibly have anticipated?

The only other major career advice I have received goes as follows: 'There are only four basic rules of medicine – never apologise, never call anyone sir, never run anywhere, and never under any circumstances miss your lunch.'

Incidentally, if you ever get to sit down to a meal with a doctor in your company, watch how he eats. They will always finish long before anybody else. This interesting approach to self nourishment stems from a simple practical necessity. In our early years after qualification mealtimes offered but a brief respite from the rigours of the day, but were prey to constant interruptions – the bleep, the telephone, other doctors wanting to talk to you about the latest miracle of human healing they had just been party to . . .

So it's not surprising that you learn to eat as fast as you can, not bothering to speak unless absolutely necessary or indulge in too many of the social graces. This therefore goes a long way to explaining why so many of us fail to develop anything approaching civilised behaviour.

The habit survives – in me, at least – until this day, along with an addiction to nicotine and black coffee. If you did not stop for a quick fix of each, you would never stop at all.

Around midnight, one weekend on call during the aforementioned job, a patient in his mid-forties was admitted under my care having had a heart attack. I was by this stage confident enough to deal with him myself and not disturb my registrar who had been up all the previous night with a particularly difficult case. If anyone deserved a good night's rest, it was he.

The fact that I had not slept for forty-eight hours was irrelevant. It was all part of the job – deal with the new admissions as best you are able and let your superiors sleep when they can. They will have more than served their dues in the past.

In those days, unlike now, the most junior doctor in the hospital looked after the intensive care unit during the night, summoning assistance only if they felt it was absolutely necessary. The patient, Mr Phillips, was duly settled on the ward and I thought gratefully of my bed, whose acquaintance I was keen to re-establish. I was just nodding off in the sister's office when she gently prodded me.

I sat up with a start.

'Go and get some sleep, Mike, while you can,' she said understandingly. 'But before you do, Mr Phillips' family have just arrived. Do you think you could have a word with them?'

I rubbed my eyes and wandered blearily down to the small sitting room where Mr Phillips' wife and parents were waiting for me. They rose as I entered.

'How is he, doctor?' asked his wife, a fair-haired, fatigued looking woman in her late thirties. 'Is he going to be all right?'

'He's fine, at the moment,' I replied, as reassuringly as I could. A man in his forties with a heart attack always presents an uncertain future. 'You can go and see him, if you like.'

'Is he out of danger?' asked his mother in a faint voice.

One thing I learned early in my career is that you can lie unmitigatedly to patients or tell them the blunt truth as best you see it, but in general it is wisest to do neither. The best approach is probably to gently blur the edges, trying to blend a cautious mix of optimism and realism.

The truth in this case was that he might die at any moment, and his long term survival prospects were bleak.

'I have to be honest with you,' I said (always a good line, that), 'the next twenty-four hours are going to be difficult.'

This was of course completely true, although I did not at that moment realise just how difficult they were going to be. What I did not say was that the twenty-four hours after that might be a bit problematical too. 'We must all just wait and see what we can do,' I reassured them.

It really does help – and I do not mean this to sound quite as cynical as it might – if relatives of patients who are potentially seriously ill feel that we are all pulling together. Like many GPs, who by and large wish fervently to retain their independence despite the prevailing attitudes of our times, we often project the idea of us all being a team for the benefit of our charges, even if we truly feel we are in fact a collection of individuals with just occasionally a common goal.

Mr Phillips' mother clasped my hand in both of hers.

'Thank you *so* much, doctor,' she said. 'We do know that you are doing all you can.'

I extricated myself gently from her clutches, promising to keep them fully informed, and crawled down the corridor and up the stairs to my bed. My glorious, wonderful, welcoming bed. We had been apart for too long, and greeted each other rapturously.

All doctors will tell you that the most difficult time to re-awake is within the first few minutes of falling asleep. In general, when the phone rings after several hours of restful repose I am awake, alert and responsive by the end of the second ring.

On occasions such as this, however, I have a recurring dream. It is always a fire engine, driving round and round the perimeter of my bed, and I wonder why it cannot just get on with the job it is designed for and leave me to my well-earned slumbers.

This time its circuit became closer and closer, until it drew to a halt on my pillow. One of the firemen got out and started tugging urgently on my shoulder.

'Mike, Mike. Wake up, Mike, I'm sorry but we need you.'

I climbed through the layers of sleep and sat up, rubbing my eyes.

'Bloody firemen,' I mumbled. 'What do you need me for? Can't you just put out the fire yourself and ring me when it's all over?'

'And what have you been taking?' asked the ward sister, regarding me good-humouredly. 'I'm sorry Mike, when you've just gone to bed, but it's Mr Phillips. He's developed an arrhythmia,' (that is an irregular beat of the heart) 'and isn't looking too good.' She paused and looked down at me again. 'Nice pyjamas,' she added sardonically.

I did not stop to dress – not because I'm an exhibitionist but mainly because I had not actually stopped to undress prior to collapsing into bed – but ran down to the ward, crumpled and fatigue-ridden as I was.

Mr Phillips looked awful, and his heart was behaving in a worryingly erratic fashion. I knew precisely what to do.

It's just that the problem was, I did not precisely do it.

What I should have done was put 200 mg of the drug I needed into 400 ml of drip solution and run it into a vein over twenty minutes. Unfortunately what I actually did was put 400 mg into 200 ml – a small matter of eight times the required concentration – and gave it to Mr Phillips without a second thought.

I went to see his family, pale and anxiously waiting, to reassure them that all was well, for the time being. They were immensely grateful for all that I was doing.

'Thank you *so* much, doctor,' said Mr Phillips' mother again. 'We do *so* appreciate – '

She got no further.

'Mike . . . Mike!' came the urgent shout from the ward. I rushed back. Mr Phillips' heartbeat had dropped to less than twenty beats a minute, his breathing was laboured and rasping, and his life hung in the balance.

'I don't understand it,' I said quietly to the sister, waiting expectantly by my side. 'It's always worked before. 400 mg in 200 ml, just as . . .'

The awful truth of what I had done struck me like a freight train. 'Oh my God,' I muttered. 'I've given him too much.'

Fatigue suddenly gone, I worked feverishly for five minutes. Sometimes, when you least expect it, knowledge comes flooding back into your mind. Half-forgotten medical facts crystallise into certainty and working on autopilot you know, you just know, that you are doing the right thing at the right time.

Mr Phillips did not respond. There was no more that I could do, and I prepared myself for the inevitable. The ward sister, older, wiser and vastly more experienced than myself, propelled me gently away from the door, closing it firmly behind her.

'Go and see his family, Mike,' she said, resting her hands on my shoulders, 'but don't say anything yet. Just say he's taken a turn for the worse, and let them come in.'

I raised my eyes to the ceiling. 'But I did it,' I said desperately. 'It's my fault. How do I tell them that?'

'You don't, not yet. They've got enough to cope with at the moment. If you unburden yourself to them now it may make you feel better, but it sure as hell won't help them at all. Trust me, I've seen it all so many times before. Do as I say, I promise you it's the right thing to do. The inquests will wait until the morning. Now go and do your job – for their sake, not your own.'

I went and saw the family.

'I have to tell you,' I said slowly, ' that he's taken a turn for the worse.' I closed my eyes and took a deep breath. 'It happens, sometimes. His heart just hasn't been able to cope with the damage.'

There was a shocked silence.

'Is he going to die?' asked his wife quietly. 'Tell us the truth, doctor, please just tell us the truth.'

The irony of this did not escape me.

'I think he may well do,' I said soberly. 'I've done all I can, given him everything I can think of, but I fear it may not be enough. Please, do go through and sit with him now, if you would like.'

They were still so grateful for my efforts, and thanked me again for all I had done. The feeling at that moment, being thanked for making the most horrendous mistake that was about to kill a husband, a son and a father, still now occasionally surfaces when things go wrong.

My first real mistake, my first death. The first occupant of the graveyard I was to acquire. I walked down the corridor to get a coffee.

All part of the job, I told myself bitterly. The sad reality of life is that in a doctor's career it will happen to each and every one of us, sooner or later, and the fact that we mostly learn to survive the experience was of no help at all, at the time.

I finished my coffee and returned leaden-footed to the ward. As

I re-entered Mr Phillips' room he was sitting up, smiling. I looked at the monitor, unable to understand what had happened. His heart was beating regularly, beautifully, wonderfully regularly. His family were chattering excitedly together by his side, laughing with relief.

I could not believe what I was seeing. I must be dreaming. I rubbed my eyes and looked again. It must be fatigue, surely it was just fatigue. But still his heart beat normally, and beat on, and still they all sat, and smiled, and rejoiced.

The antidote had worked, and he had recovered. He left hospital four days later and as far as I know lives on to this day, but all I can remember is that I made a horrible mistake which nearly killed him. I was tired beyond exhaustion, overworked beyond reason, and staggering under the weight of responsibility I had insufficient experience to deal with, but still that was no excuse.

A man had almost died because of my actions. It is an experience you never forget.

I never said anything about what had happened, and I am sure neither Mr Phillips nor his family ever knew. In truth I had desperately wanted to tell them, to unburden myself from the guilt, but as the ward sister said later that night, 'If you don't tell them today, you can still tell them tomorrow. But if you do let them know what went on you can't retract it when it suits you. It's called medicine, Mike, and you haven't been around long enough yet to understand how it all works. But you will, one day you will.'

She was right then and remains right, I believe, to this day. Would I do the same again now, twenty years later?

Probably.

A week later I received a letter from Mr Phillips' wife.

'We just wanted to thank you for saving Ian's life,' she wrote. 'We have so much to thank you for. In our hour of need you were there, and we will never forget it. Thank you *so* much, doctor. You were so wonderful, in our hour of need.'

I still have the letter tucked away, but I have never read it since that day. There is no need. I know each and every word of it by heart.

The following happened later in the same job. I was still making my way precariously through an ever enlarging medical minefield, a very junior physician in a very large hospital in the spectral wastes of Cumbria. I had now progressed beyond the worrying stage when you are uncertain which end of the stethoscope you insert into your ears, and had forsaken all those other uses for the rubbery bits. Not only was I now considered fit to be let loose upon society, but also to lead others more innocent and inexperienced than I into one of the perpetual medical cul-de-sacs I seemed forever to be finding myself in.

In other words I had a medical student with me, and I was supposed to be teaching him.

It was not quite so much the blind leading the blind as the terribly uncertain leading the inquisitively eager. But I was coping – I was better able to survive chronic sleep deprivation than he, and had more letters after my name. More importantly I had spent more of my formative years in the pub, and would no longer get drunk on two pints of lager top. David – my 'student' – needed only so much as to sniff half a shandy before he would start wobbling down the corridors.

It made me feel so superior, and so much in control.

We were called to casualty one day – well, David was called and I followed meekly along to see if I could learn something. The patient was middle-aged, thin, balding and in pain. I had not a clue what was wrong with him, but I had one significant advantage. He was naked, save for one of those beautifully tailored hospital robes with ties at the back that never quite do up, and I was fully clothed.

These things matter. He would have believed anything I told him.

Back in the early 1980s – and this is not being politically-incorrect, just statistically accurate – there were many doctors practising in the country who were not necessarily born within the confines of the United Kingdom. In my first hospital, to my surprise, I was the only English doctor on the staff. I wasn't in fact entirely sure from where all the others originated – we couldn't always understand each other, for a start – but as many of the patients were non-Caucasian themselves it was me who was frequently left in the dark. Medically, I expected it. Linguistically it came as a bit of a shock.

The problem had arisen due to a transient shortage of British doctors. The government of the day decided to import a large number of replacements from abroad, while increasing the student intake to medical schools in the apparently sensible hope that within five years the problem would be resolved.

There was, however, one small point they neglected to take into account. Their great plan – no doubt the culmination of years of expense-account lunches – relied upon all the imported doctors meekly going home again. But they didn't.

Hence, five years later, there was a glut of young British doctors with no jobs available for them. They began to go abroad . . .

I digress.

In the hospital where I was working, there was a very Welsh surgeon named Dai Davies. The Welsh are generally highly original with their nomenclature – I once came across a gynae-cologist called William William Williams.

Having seen my prospective patient in casualty I decided that whatever his pathology, it was not within my remit to resolve – he needed a surgeon, not a physician as had initially been thought. Communication is an art, not a science, which may explain why so many doctors are completely lacking in this most important of skills.

'I'm sorry, Mr Slater,' I said carelessly, 'but I shall have to ask one of my colleagues to see to you. If you'd like to wait here . . .'

He sat up abruptly, looking worried.

'What's wrong with me, doctor? Can you tell me what's going to happen now?'

It can be very difficult to reassure an agitated patient when you are young, inexperienced and short of time. I decided therefore not to bother.

'Just wait here, Mr Slater, and I'll have somebody with you shortly,' I said impatiently and turned to leave, closing the curtains around him.

'Is that it?' whispered David in my ear, obviously wondering if I was ever going to teach him something medical.

'Yes,' I replied. 'Can't do anything more for this one. We'll just have to leave him to Dai.'

We were walking off down the corridor, white coats flowing imperiously in our wake and Mr Slater forgotten, when there was a commotion behind us, a clattering of wheels and somebody shouting pitifully.

'Doctor, doctor,' I could hear behind us, growing ominously closer.

I hastened my steps, hoping I could slip around the nearest corner before becoming involved in a situation that clearly had nothing to do with me, but then 'Doctor, doctor – you in front of me, walking away – *doctor*!'

There was to be no escape.

I turned around and stopped, open-mouthed. Mr Slater was hobbling down the corridor towards us, drip stand trailing in his wake with his hospital tunic flying open, his pathology clearly exposed for all to see. Intrigued visitors and staff lined the walls of the corridor, following his progress. This was much more interesting than coming to see Auntie Mabel in the geriatric unit.

He stumbled and fell, the drip stand tumbling on top of him. I groaned in sympathy.

'Don't leave me,' he called pathetically, waving a hand in our direction.

I resisted the temptation to murmur, 'But we've only just met,' and waited for what was to come next.

'Don't do this to me,' he called feebly. 'You can't just leave me to die . . .'

It's a funny feeling, sitting in the pub, having a drink and reflecting.

That is to say, it's a funny feeling reflecting in the pub, not sitting in the pub having a drink because that to a young doctor is as natural as breathing, only slightly more expensive. The pub is as essential to the life of a medical student as. . . . well, as the juke box and the fruit machine.

Fruit machines once used to be a lucrative source of income to the impoverished, or at least, the proper old-fashioned ones which still had fruit on were. Oh, the joy of seeing those three lemons, or a couple of cherries.

One day, purely by chance – no self respecting student would ever deliberately waste a drink in such a manner – I knocked over a pint of Young's finest as it rested on top of the glorious machine in the pub close to the medical school. We all know the truly beneficial effects of alcohol upon the human body, but the effect upon this particular fruit machine was equally wonderful to behold. Fruit machines, like students, need lubricating on a regular basis, but equally like medical students the effect upon them can be hard to predict. In the case of this particular fruit machine the booze made it malfunction, so much so in fact, that it forgot how to take our money . . .

Each time we pressed the start button – and we pressed it sub-sequently quite a lot of times that evening – the wheels continued to spin until a winning line came into view. Then chink, chink, chink, and out it paid. We emptied the machine just as last orders were called, which seemed to us an entirely satisfactory state of affairs.

Students subsidise their way through medical school by a

variety of means – some by actually working (honestly), some by subjecting themselves to the pleasures of medical experimentation on new drugs – good money, but often acutely uncomfortable and entailing alarming side effects – and some by organised crime.

My flatmate and I simply toured London and poured pints of Young's bitter down the back of fruit machines for six months, until word spread and they withdrew that particular type of ready income. A sad day that was too, but it was great fun while it lasted.

For the first two years as a student, I naïvely believed that students drank, but doctors did not. This touching faith in the sanctity of our professional superiors lasted until I actually met a doctor in a pub, and realised they drank an equivalent amount, if not even more, the only difference being that they could afford it.

My first experience at close hand of the hold that alcohol exerts on the medical profession was during my anaesthetics attachment at a well known hospital in Reading. I was bleeped by the on-call anaesthetist at ten o'clock one evening. When I met him it struck me immediately that he looked staggeringly like Mark Knopfler – lead guitarist and vocalist of the rock band Dire Straits, for the uninitiated – only more laid back.

In fact given his generally laid-back approach to anaesthetics I think it probably was Mark Knopfler, early on his first career.

'Got an appendectomy,' he said, casually looking at his watch. 'Half an hour – plenty of time for last orders.'

We strolled down to the operating theatre, met the young man who was about to be parted from his appendix, and Mark duly anaesthetised him. Ten thirty, and time was running out, I thought.

I had so much to learn.

'How long will you be, John?' Mark asked the surgeon.

'Twenty-five minutes, thereabouts.'

'Good,' said Mark happily, 'time for a quick couple, then. Come on Mike, hurry up now.'

I must have looked surprised – oh, the innocence of youth – because he laid a hand on my shoulder and said gently, 'Pub. Drink. Now.'

'But . . . what about the patient?' I asked pathetically.

'Oh, he won't mind. He's asleep and John'll give us a shout if there's a problem. OK, John?'

'OK,' came the reply. 'Bring us a pint, will you? Got a tricky laparotomy coming up after this.'

My conscience was troubling me. Leave theatre with the anaesthetist but without the anaesthetised? It took a bit of thought, as much as three or four seconds, and then we were off, heading for the pub.

Mark Knopfler and I had a couple of beers completely oblivious to whatever was happening in theatre, and after twenty-five minutes of idle relaxation wandered back to our now appendixless patient, whereupon Mr Knopfler woke him up. Not one single person seemed to think there was anything in the least untoward about this whole event.

To return to where I was – in the pub, reflecting.

It is a sad but true fact of life that no doctor is capable of indulging in conversation with a colleague (I have heard it said that no doctor is actually capable of indulging in normal conversation with anyone at all) without mentioning his car, his privately educated children, his last round of golf and how well he played that tricky shot at the thirteenth, or how good the skiing was last year at some place in Austria you've never heard of and what fun they had with the mulled wine after that second glass.

If you survive this dreary preamble you can move on to the really interesting stuff. The conversation inevitably turns to patients and the innumerable indignities they suffer as we try to pretend we know what we are doing whilst all the time wondering why people think we want to even look at their haemorrhoids, let alone touch them.

Have you ever heard a six-year-old say, 'When I grow up I want to perform barium enemas for a living'? Not while there are still trains to be driven and sweet shops to run you won't.

There is a warm comforting feeling about reflecting on the vagaries of life's inhumanity to others whilst downing your third pint of Theakstone's Old Peculiar. You can be reasonably sure that there will be at least one story within the first quarter of an hour involving orifices, the unusual objects variously removed from them, and how many people it took. (Yes, I have once been in theatre when a vibrator was surgically removed from the dark recesses of a patient's colon, and it was still buzzing.)

The surreal nature of the world we inhabit suddenly struck me one evening as I was recounting the tale of a memorable patient I encountered as a junior physician. I have never had the pleasure of meeting the fattest man in the world but I did once enjoy a brief acquaintance with the fattest man in a Midlands town that had best remain nameless.

One of my friends, Paul, had kindly volunteered to cover an early evening stint for me whilst I attended some now long-forgotten function. I duly returned – surprisingly sober for two o'clock in the morning – to finish off the night's entertainment. My amiable colleague greeted me with an expression of mixed anguish and controlled amusement – the former due to a newly acquired double hernia, the latter from that divine pleasure that only ever occurs when you know you have a problem which is almost completely without solution but which is just about to become somebody else's responsibility.

'Interesting patient in ward three, Mike,' said Paul with a glint of something demonic in his eyes. 'Worth taking a look at.'

'Which bed?' I asked innocently.

He considered a moment.

'Beds two, three and four,' he answered cryptically, and limped off down the corridor in search of the most comfortable truss the nurses' home could provide. I had intended to go straight to bed, but nobody could ignore such a situation and continue to call himself a junior doctor with any degree of pride.

As usual at this hour the hospital was in almost complete silence. There were the usual nocturnal sounds – an odd snore, the occasional groan and some intermittent hacking coughs (no, not the patients, but the highly trained on-call surgical team playing three card brag in the casualty department). As I entered ward three all was in darkness save for the last three cubicles, at the end of which stood several nurses, the medical registrar and the night porter, all assuming various poses of perplexed curiosity.

I wandered slowly down to join them, wondering what I was about to find, and peeked round the curtain. Inside the cubicle lay the largest man I have ever seen. Lengthwise he was pretty average, but in girth he was something special. His vast folds of cold, clammy fat flowed down each side of the bed, supported to some degree by the simple expedient of piling all the unused linen on the floor either side of him.

He had been completely beyond the scope of any weighing machine the hospital could provide, but it was thought he weighed in at around forty-eight stone. I have not the least idea how he got from where he had been to where he now was, but could only assume that some ingenious soul had managed to negotiate a JCB down the hospital corridors, being no doubt eternally thankful that the ward was on the ground floor.

'What's wrong with him?' I hissed to the harassed registrar.

'Pretty much everything,' he responded. 'Surgeons say he's got a strangulated hernia . . .'

'The obstetricians think it's sextuplets,' murmured a young Irish nurse in my ear, trying unsuccessfully to stifle a giggle.

'. . . but they won't operate,' continued the registrar, flashing her a look of stern disapproval (no sense of humour, some doctors), 'because they say he has no chance of surviving an anaesthetic. He's got heart failure, kidney damage, diabetes . . .'

'Trench foot, ingrowing toenails and hairy ears,' whispered the Irish nurse, barely perceptibly. I warmed to her instantly.

'. . . and very soon he is going to die,' finished the registrar. 'He's been brought here to do it.'

'Why us?' I asked.

'Firstly, because we're the on-call physicians, secondly because they brought him in through the french windows and couldn't get him out through the door of the ward to anywhere else,' came the answer. 'And thirdly this is the only ward in the hospital with three consecutive empty cubicles available.'

We stood there for some time, wondering what – or what not – we might do, and then gradually drifted away. For once I managed to get some sleep, waking the next morning – Saturday – to find much to my surprise that the patient was still alive, though barely so. He continued to survive throughout the rest of the day despite our complete inability to do anything more than make him as comfortable as we could.

I retired to bed that night with him still precariously clinging to existence.

At 3 a.m. he was clinging no more, and I was called to certify his death. It is generally a tiresome task to be awoken from well-earned repose to certify a fact that several nurses have already conclusively proved by the simple expedient of noting the patient is no longer breathing. Tradition, however, demands that we should shamble bleary-eyed on to the ward, mumble, 'Yep, he's dead,' then shamble away again into the black hole from which he had emerged.

The exercise was made all the more bearable by the continued presence of the Irish nurse, who had obviously thought a step or two ahead of the rest of us.

'What are we going to do with him now?' she asked, rolling her eyes deliciously.

'Move him to . . .' I stopped.

Moving forty-eight stone of living humanity must have been

pretty tough. Moving forty-eight stone of recently expired carcass did not bear thinking about.

An hour later, the entire complement of junior doctors on night duty in the hospital, together with two porters and a very helpful chap who had wandered into casualty with a fishhook in his left thigh (no, don't ask), stood outside the mortuary with our recently departed charge spread-eagled across the three hospital beds we had joined together with rolled up sheets as his temporary mode of transport.

There remained one problem. We couldn't get him in through the mortuary door. Not only that, but the mortuary was at the bottom of a long and gentle slope from the hospital itself and we were completely unable to get him back up the hill to anywhere else. Exhaustion was but another shove or two away.

As dawn threatened to break the situation had deteriorated.

We had manoeuvred him off the beds, on to the ground and into the doorway, and there we were. Stuck. He was jammed irrevocably between the uprights, large rolls of adipose tissue cascading down either side of the creaking timbers. No amount of pushing, prodding, heaving or tugging could change the predicament we were in.

What made all this worse was that the mortuary was right next to the main gates of the hospital. As we all knew only too well, in just an hour or two's time the daily influx of visitors would be passing within a few yards of where we stood, sweating, exhausted and beginning to be overtaken by intractable fits of insane giggling.

I honestly don't know what we would have done had the Irish nurse not had a brother, who happened to be a builder, who happened to be working on a building site near by. Not only that, but as good fortune would have it he just happened to be at home, asleep and sharing a flat with another Irish builder working on the same site who even more fortuitously turned out to be a crane driver.

Just imagine for a while, if you can, the sight of a crane demolishing the entrance to a mortuary, lifting a forty-eight stone dead man into the back of a pick-up truck and rumbling off into the early morning sunrise as we threw a tarpaulin over the dusty remains of the largest man in the Midlands – just as the first visitors to the hospital appeared on the horizon and we wiped our brows in relief.

One of the sadnesses of your early career, when jobs last only six months or a year, is that you meet, get to know and then quickly lose contact with so many of your peers. It is a shifting, changing world and you survive as best you can.

Wasu, whose full name I never knew and would probably never have been able to pronounce, was a strikingly handsome Pakistani casualty officer with a tremendous sense of fun and a wickedly mischievous smile. He was a perfect gentleman, and all the nurses and patients adored him. A well-respected gynaecologist in his own country, he had a sister who ran a hospital in Pakistan; she had dispatched him to England to acquire an English degree, without which – at that time – he could apparently not obtain consultant status in the land of his birth.

He took a humble casualty job, far below his undoubted abilities, and studied diligently in his spare time. His one weakness was for Bacardi and Coke, a drink I was initially unfamiliar with but which by force of circumstance I soon came to know and love. This was aided and abetted in no small measure by the happy coincidence of a cousin of Wasu's owning a delicatessen in the town near by, and being an exporter of Bacardi to Pakistan on the side. We were blessed with an inexhaustible supply, and it would have been churlish not to have taken advantage of it.

The hospital rota often threw us together on 'crash' duty. At any significant emergency – for example a cardiac arrest or a sudden collapse – the designated doctors of the day, who each carried a special 'arrest' bleep, would be summoned to the site of the emergency, immediately discarding all other duties. It presented a series of wonderful opportunities to speed down the long hospital corridors through the crowds of visitors and hospital staff, white coats flowing in our wake, looking as if we were both really important and completely in control of what we were doing.

Wasu kept a specially adapted halo in his pocket that he would don at a moment's notice when such a duty called. I once even saw him turn up to a sudden death with an 'I am a hero' sandwich board draped over his body, front and back. When bored – or to be more truthful when bored and with several Bacardis under our belts – Wasu would tap me on the shoulder at an unguarded moment and whisper, 'Three, two, one . . . go!' before bellowing 'Cardiac arrest' at the top of his voice.

Soon we would be sprinting the length of the hospital, shouting, 'Clear the way, emergency doctors in a hurry,' before collapsing giggling out of sight at the end of our journey. Yes, I do know it is childish, but we worked very hard and this was just our moment or two of light entertainment.

One afternoon we were sitting having coffee in the doctors' common room – with a hint of Bacardi, just a hint – when the arrest bleep went off and the message came over the hospital tannoy. 'Arrest team to casualty, arrest team to casualty, arrest team . . .'

We rose in unison, and ran.

The arrest bleep would go off maybe three or four times a week, and we might find any of a range of scenarios on arrival at our destination. Sometimes a nurse had just panicked and we found an embarrassed patient sitting up in bed wondering what all the emergency staff were doing disturbing their afternoon's sleep. On other occasions there might be a death we could do nothing about, and sometimes a real life or death emergency when the adrenaline flowed and we all pulled together to endeavour to save the life of the patient.

We were not, sadly, always destined to succeed, but we always did the very best that we could with whatever situation we found on our arrival.

On this particular afternoon we sprinted down the corridors in our usual light-hearted fashion and slid to a halt on the polished floors of the casualty department. The waiting area was normally a busy metropolis of the injured, the curious, the malingerers, the socially deprived and the hangers-on looking for a free cup of coffee and a place to sit undisturbed for a couple of hours (or the best part of a day, if they chose their time right).

Today was different, and I remember it vividly. There was blood everywhere. Patients, staff and visitors alike lined the wall, shocked and silent. Wasu, quicker to react than I, spoke tersely to the nearest two nurses.

'Where's the patient?' he asked.

The two nurses pointed to adjoining cubicles, unable to speak. Wasu murmured under his breath.

'OK, Mike, let's see what we've got. You take the one on the left, and I'll take the one on the right.'

We walked soberly across the department, wondering what awaited us. I pulled back the curtain in my allotted cubicle, stepped inside and turned to face my patient. What met my eyes was beyond my initial comprehension.

Part of a torso lay before me. The body had been severed in half just below the navel, and I had from the waist down. I stood and looked for a moment, unable fully to take in what I could see. Gradually my reeling senses cleared and I began to take stock of the situation.

Outside the cubicle I could sense a growing expectation. We were the doctors, the 'arrest team'. We were expected to be *doing* something. But to do what, precisely?

'Pssst,' I heard from the next-door cubicle. It was Wasu. 'What have you got in there, Mike?'

'The bottom half of a body,' I whispered back. 'What about you?'

'Top half,' he returned. There was a short silence and then he added urgently, 'What the hell are we supposed to do?'

To explain, we later learned that the neatly divided body belonged to a recently bankrupted local businessman who had decided to commit suicide by the simple – and brutally efficient – expedient of lying across the nearest available railway track in front of an oncoming train. He had been sliced clinically in two, and a fleet of ambulances on arriving at the scene, miraculously thinking they could feel a pulse, had brought him into casualty – one ambulance bringing the head part, another the bottom.

A third was left to seek the poor man's left hand, which remained undiscovered at the scene.

Two stretchers, two cubicles and two doctors, without a clue what to do.

We were both aware of the growing unrest beyond our curtains, and I knew we couldn't stay hidden with our respective half corpses for ever. Something had to be done, and fairly soon. I came to a sudden decision.

Even now I cannot fully justify what I did, but it was all I could think of, under the circumstances.

'It's OK, Wasu, I've got an idea,' I hissed. 'Step out of the cubicle when I say "Go."'

'What have you got in mind?' he countered uncertainly.

'Trust me,' I said. 'I'm a doctor. Three, two, one . . .'

Our audience awaited expectantly. We stepped outside, Wasu wondering what was to come. I rubbed my hands briskly together and clapped him firmly on his shoulder.

'Well, doctor,' I said jovially, 'I've got the bottom half working. How are you doing with the head and the neck?'

You could have heard the proverbial pin drop, and then drop again. Wasu looked aghast. The casualty sister, a diminutive Scot with a forceful personality and a previously unrealised intimate acquaintance with the Marquess of Queensberry rules, strode across the waiting room and slapped me firmly across the face.

'In all mai years,' she spluttered, 'in all mai years as a nurse, I have never, ever heard something so insensitive uttered in the name of medicine.'

Silence reigned, nobody knowing how to act. And then one of the casualty nurses started laughing, tentatively at first and then in an uncontrolled fashion, and slowly, but surely, the rest of the occupants of the casualty department – patients, staff and visitors alike – joined in.

You encounter some weird and wonderful, some surreal and bizarre situations in a career in medicine and learn how to adjust, how to take them in your stride.

But as we stood outside those curtains, our corpse concealed within, my cheek stinging and the slap echoing in my ears, with a waiting room full of complete strangers laughing almost hysterically, I knew that somehow it would never become more surreal than this.

8

A Little Trouble in South America (Part 1)

Time has passed. It is now some fifteen years since the events I am about to relate took place. The provisions of the Statute of Limitations must surely apply by now. I hope . . .

After all, starting a riot in a brothel in Central America where the doorman sometime later had his head blown off with a double-barrelled shotgun is not so very terrible a crime.

Is it?

It had all begun six months earlier in a lunch queue in the officers' mess at RAF St Athan, an engineering station in South Wales. I had joined the air force on a short service commission (five years and counting) some eighteen months previously, and this was my second posting.

My first was at RAF Chivenor, a fighter pilot training station in North Devon, had been negotiated with just a minor blot or two on an ever enlarging copybook, but here already the dark storm clouds were beginning to gather ominously on the horizon.

For a start, the Senior Medical Officer (SMO) and I just did not get on. A dour Scot with obsessive compulsive tendencies that to my mind bordered on the certifiable, he was unable to cope with my rather more carefree approach to life, and tensions frequently ran high.

'You didn't want to go to the Falklands, did you?' he asked with an odd expression on his face – the one that heralded his 'I am about to tell you something you are not going to like but which I am going to enjoy enormously' announcements. Of his four junior doctors, I was indisputably his least favourite.

'Is that a rhetorical question?' I asked, adding maliciously, 'Sorry, rhetorical – it means – '

'I know what it means,' he snapped back, irritated. Moral victory to me – if he was going to give me some bad news, I wanted to make sure he derived the least possible pleasure from it. 'Anyway, you're not going to the Falklands for four months because you're off to Belize for six, instead,' he finished triumphantly.

Several immediate responses came to mind, Why? being one of them, followed by When?, Who With?, and What for? Not to mention the one I had no intention of yet admitting to, namely, so where the bloody hell is Belize, then?

He was awaiting my reaction, confidently expecting it to be unfavourable.

'Belize,' I said thoughtfully, stroking my chin. 'That's one of those new stations just north of Birmingham, isn't it?'

When I first applied to join the air force, tours abroad for us part-timers – doctors on a short service commission of five years – were pretty much out of the question. Unless, that is, you wanted to spend three years in expatriate isolation in Germany playing silly war games on a regular basis, and I, for one, did not. And as if that was not bad enough, can you imagine not only losing to the German football team but having to live there at the same time?

Then along came the Falklands, and everything changed.

Once the islands were retaken, troops had to be stationed there to hang on to them, and troops needed doctors. Which was unfortunate, really, because none of us doctors needed the Falklands. I personally would rather have spent my four months sitting in a dentist's waiting room whilst in need of a couple of root fillings.

The upshot was that we all had to go somewhere, unaccompanied (phew, the relief), and four months with the penguins was seen by most as positively benign compared with six months in the jungle with the mosquitoes, the tarantulas, the coral snakes . . . and the Grenadier Guards.

'I'm going to Belize,' I announced carelessly, on arriving home.

'Is that one of those new stations just north of Birmingham?' asked my wife.

'Close,' I said, 'but it might help if I told you it was a bit south of Mexico.'

'Mexico Wolverhampton?'

'And north of Brazil,' I added.

'Oh,' she said, reflecting. 'That Belize, then. What should I pack?'

'My suitcase,' I suggested.

'No, I meant for me. What should I pack to wear?'

'Um, nothing,' I replied, grimacing.

'Oh, it's that sort of place, is it?' she said, her eyes narrowing. 'And I always thought the RAF were so conservative in their habits.'

'They are,' I said slowly, 'and I've no idea what sort of place it is, except that it's not a "We're going" sort of place at all. More an "I'm going and I'm afraid that you're staying behind" sort of place.'

'I see,' she said, tight-lipped. 'It's like that, is it?'

And it was.

I was summoned to see the RAF hierarchy up in Huntingdon prior to my departure, to be interviewed by a strange dinosaur of a creature I had long thought to be extinct.

A senior RAF doctor with a sense of humour.

'Ah, Sparrow,' he said waving carelessly at the chair in front of his desk. 'Take a seat – got a memo about you here, somewhere. In fact . . .' he pursed his lips, '. . . I've got quite a few memos about you, come to think of it. Still,' he continued, smiling amiably, 'we'll disregard all but the most recent, shall we?'

I looked at the pile of memos in his left hand, and the single one in his right. 'Disregarding looks like a pretty good idea to me, sir.'

'Thought you might be in agreement,' he said, flicking idly through some of the papers in front of him. 'Interesting career you've had, young man. I see it was you who . . .' He caught himself, and came back to the point in hand. 'Off to Belize, I see. Know where it is, by any chance?'

'I do now, sir,' I said, feeling slightly unnerved. Two minutes in the same room with an officer more than two ranks above my own, and no hint of a reprimand. It was all rather confusing.

'Two things you need to know,' he said, leaning across his desk. 'All the Belizians want to do is lie in the sun all day drinking beer and then make love to each other. My advice to you is don't get in the way of either of them.'

And that was my pre-tour briefing in its entirety, although I have paraphrased the odd word.

And bloody good advice it was too.

You step off the tarmac in England on a cold, damp, grey January morning, and fifteen hours later emerge from the plane at Belize airport – one concrete strip and a man with a megaphone – into a wall of heat and humidity that hits you like a sledgehammer.

A few people are meeting friends and colleagues, or people returning from leave, and somewhere out there is a doctor waiting to greet me before going home on the plane I have just arrived on, his six-month sentence complete. But right now all I want to do is be able to breathe without setting my lungs on fire. I stand around gasping, waiting for the air-conditioned bus to come and drive me to the mess, and eventually it arrives . . .

But they've left the air-conditioning behind.

A short journey later we reach the officers' mess, which at first sight is a disappointment – at second a disaster. It appears to be little more than a tiny bar with a concrete floor and an extended veranda covered by an atap – a local wooden construction with a roof of dried-out palm leaves.

Beyond that, the dark green Nissen huts which are the accommodation blocks lie scattered amongst the scrubland and the trees. Home, for the next six months.

My heart was already beginning to sink.

But it grew on you.

The heat, the jungle, the absence of anything approaching real work . . . The mosquitoes, the iguanas, the fact that the bar stayed open until the last person was unconscious, all of these things I soon came to know and love. As I write these words I can imagine myself back there once more, and allow myself to miss it, for a while.

Life soon settled into a routine. Each day you would awake and wander bleary-eyed into the warmth of the early morning sun. I had just missed the rainy season, with its furious bursts of tropical downpours at but a moment's notice. Six months of almost unadulterated sunshine stretched ahead, interspersed by the occasional torrential midday thunderstorm from which you dried out in a matter of moments.

I would sit on the bank outside my room, taking it all in before diving for cover from the thick clouds of acrid smoke which heralded the arrival of the mosquito sprayers, a twice daily ritual. I always thought any right-minded mozzy would have seen them coming by now – 'Spraying time, boys. Let's make ourselves scarce for a while,' only to return twenty minutes later when the fug had died down, baying for the blood of an Englishman.

I suppose mosquitoes just aren't that intelligent – along with some of the army officers, who would sit through the smoke without any apparent discomfort.

Next I would greet Iggy – original name that – my adopted iguana, a huge, striking-looking male who patrolled his territory just outside my door. We would sit and pass the time of day together, me watching him do . . . well, nothing at all, really.

Breakfast, a leisurely affair, soon followed, and then it was off to what passed for a morning surgery. The army doctor, a colonel who outranked me by some degree, saw the army patients, and the RAF doctor – i.e. myself – saw whatever the small contingent of air force personnel could provide . . . generally one to four people, plus the odd dog or cat.

After that, the day was largely your own, and you passed it as best you could. Backgammon, a cut-throat variety of Ludo whose name now escapes me but in which blatant cheating was not so much accepted as fervently encouraged, reading, writing the odd letter, and most arduous of all deciding precisely where to position your sun-lounger in order to avoid having to get up and move it at less than three-hour intervals as the sun dawdled lazily across the cloudless sky.

Oh, how we suffered. And yet boredom was an ever-present companion, lurking ominously beyond the patina of content.

My function in life, once morning surgery was completed, was to remain within calling distance of the helicopter squadron. Squadron 33, from Odiham, were a fine upstanding bunch of young men – or a wanton collection of sociopaths with only a loose grip on reality, according to your point of view – who flew twin-engined Pumas around the country with what at first sight seemed to be cavalier abandon, but at second supreme professionalism.

Mostly they would be moving troops and equipment from one impenetrable part of the jungle to another, but their other role was that of the emergency service. At any hour of the day or night they could be summoned to rescue casualties from the field. It was here that their undoubted expertise as pilots would shine through.

My task was to balance up the individual needs of the patient at risk against the perils of flying to whatever part of the country he might be requiring to be rescued from. The powers that be, poor deluded souls as they were, believed innocently that as I was supposed to know a little about each discipline involved I would be the best qualified person to assess whether a helicopter should be dispatched for any one incident.

In truth, I suppose I knew a smidgen more about medicine than the average helicopter pilot, and rather a lot more about negotiating a helicopter around the unforgiving Belizian terrain than any army doctor I had yet to encounter. Of all the personnel there present on the base, I was undoubtedly the best qualified.

Which doesn't half make you worry about the abilities of the rest of them . . .

Belize was then about ninety per cent covered by jungle, and finding wounded army personnel, especially at night, was by no means an easy task. Given the degree of forestation it was somewhat deficient in landmarks with which to orientate oneself, and flying with any sort of power failure was hazardous in the extreme. The first time I flew at night I was blasé about the difficulties – until we flew beyond the environs of the airstrip, the only ground source of illumination, and the pilot turned the navigation lights off.

That was the moment I understood what real flying was all about. Most of my spare time I spent sitting excitedly in the co-pilot's seat, pretending to be a pilot. Some days the helicopter even took off . . .

Flying was quite uncomplicated for us amateurs out there – lots of air space to buzz around in, very few buildings to bump into and no one to complain when you missed your landing point by a mile. For the professionals, however, it was licence to play – carte blanche to do as they pleased providing they brought the helicopter back in more or less the same shape as they had taken it out, and preferably on the same day.

It was a captivating experience. Speeding across the roof of the jungle, hovering in tiny clearings, weaving at ground level between the trees themselves in the sparser areas, and in true *Apocalypse Now* fashion skimming the clear waters of the forest-lined rivers, hopping at the last minute over the bridges . . . and just occasionally diving beneath them, heart in your mouth.

It was awesome, at times, and at last I came to understand why the pilots wore all that waterproof underwear.

My first challenge came a couple of days after my arrival in the country.

'Got a call to a plane crash,' yelled Kevin, the pilot on call, throwing me a flying suit. 'Are you up for it so soon in your stay here, or what?'

I was up for it, whatever it might be.

We flew out across the deep, deep blue sea under the cloudless sky, heading towards the bearing we had been given. For somebody who had only just disembarked into the country it all seemed unreal. I had previously flown in the fast jets at Chivenor, and on the way out Kevin gave me the rudiments of flying a helicopter. 'You just waggle this big stick around a bit,' he explained, 'and try not to press too many of the buttons.'

As we approached the area in which we expected to find the stricken plane, I clambered out of the co-pilot's seat and into the back of the helicopter, preparing to be winched down to the casualties, if any.

'Should be there in a moment,' said Kevin over the intercom a few minutes later. 'Time to start looking around.'

'What for?' I asked fatuously.

'Oh, a symphony orchestra playing the Dead March on an island,' he retorted sardonically. 'A shoal of dolphins doing a synchronised swimming number, Jacques Cousteau discovering yet another underwater Atlantis . . . How the bloody hell do I know? That, down there, is the sea,' he added sardonically. 'Just look for anything that doesn't routinely belong there.'

We found him with surprising ease. The ocean in this part of the world is full of tiny 'cays' – small islands with a single palm tree, a couple of grains of sand and room for either a helicopter pad or one out of every ten parachutists to land without eviscerating themselves upon the finest coral reef to be found outside Australia.

There is one spot far out into the sea where a sandbank rises just inches below the surface of the waves. There you can stand, alone and free, without any visible means of support, imagining that you are walking upon the water for the one and only time in your life.

And if that wasn't enough, as you return to your boat hordes of dolphins follow you back to your port, gambolling playfully in the bow wave. What more could you ask?

He was smoking a cigarette, the man we had been sent to rescue, sitting nonchalantly on his upturned aircraft which had crash landed just next to the tiniest of cays – two grains of sand and a palm leaf. More infuriatingly, as we hovered overhead he waved cheerily up to us – which resolved one pressing dilemma of the outward journey, i.e. which of us was going to be winched down there to get him out of his predicament.

'Looks pretty much OK to me,' I opined. 'All limbs moving, nice healthy colour, minimal risk of internal haemorrhage, no obvious signs of life-threatening infectious diseases . . .'

'Meaning you don't think you are the man to go down and bring him up?' asked Kevin perceptively.

'Meaning it is my first task in the country,' I corrected firmly. 'And I am not yet fully broken in. I think I should give that honour to your winch-man here. See how the professionals do it.'

So we lowered him down and watched in a detached manner as a heated argument broke out below us. There was lots of arm-waving and gnashing of teeth, and then Peter, the winch-man, was reeled in back on his own.

'He doesn't want to be rescued,' he informed us seriously. 'Says he has friends who will be along in a while and he is perfectly happy where he is, thank you very much.'

'Why on earth . . . ?' I asked, bewildered.

'Drug runner,' explained Kevin with a wink. 'They fly all their supplies into here on these two-a-penny contraptions – you often see them burnt out in the jungle. First one I've come across in the water, though – probably ran out of fuel and jettisoned all his cargo before he landed, I'd guess. Sat there waiting patiently for his friends to turn up, poor devil, and look what happens to him.' He grinned wickedly. 'Aero-medical evacuation arrives unexpectedly, and suddenly he thinks he's going to be rescued, whether he wants to or not. But he's got a surprise coming.'

'Which is?' I asked.

'We passed a police launch twenty minutes back,' continued Kevin with a chuckle. 'And there's no other boat of any sort for absolutely miles around.'

He threw the helicopter into a sharp turn, banking to the right, and started correcting his course back to base.

'So you'll just fly off and leave him there, then . . .'

'Yes,' said Kevin, and 'No,' said Peter a split second later, staring down to the waters below. 'Plane's shifted, boss. It's beginning to sink – best winch me down again.'

Our reluctant rescuee was now inching his way precariously along the bottom of the upturned fuselage towards the tail. As we watched, the nose dipped suddenly below the water, throwing the tail up in the air and nearly catapulting the pilot into the clear blue waters. He hung on desperately, waving up at us with a look of panic on his face, the water lapping his ankles.

Peter was lowered down again and returned a few minutes later with a dripping wet Sicilian-looking chap, now beaming all over his face. 'Thanks for the lift,' he enthused. 'It was getting a bit scary down there.'

'You don't seem all that worried about the loss of your plane,' I said curiously as he towelled himself dry.

He shrugged. 'I'm alive, aren't I? And besides, I can always get another plane in the morning.'

'Just like that?' I asked.

'Just like that,' boasted Paulo, as our passenger was called. 'Buy myself a couple, if I want to.'

And how do you manage that, precisely? I was wondering innocently. But there are some questions you just don't ask.

Up to this point our journey had been light-hearted and agreeable, but now some of the realities of the situation began to strike home.

We had on board a drug runner – an apparently amiable one who for the moment greatly appreciated his rescue from a rapidly sinking plane, but a drug runner, nonetheless. It was about now that he and ourselves began to have slightly differing ideas as to where we should be dropping him off.

We, of course, had on our side the helicopter in which to fly him around. But then he had his gun . . .

Originally we had thought we might either deliver him to the fast approaching police launch, or return to our base and let the Military Police take over. After all, we were flying the helicopter and up until this point had sort of thought we had the major choice in the matter. Peter and I sat regarding his gun with increasing concern.

It was aimed unerringly for Peter's chest, which I thought a little churlish given his role in our heroic rescue, but I suppose it was at least pointed in an amiable, appreciative 'Thank you very much for saving my life' sort of way. He then indicated where he would like us to drop him off, which was diametrically opposed to either of our initial intentions.

So we compromised. We flew him exactly where he wanted to go, and we all agreed what a really good idea it was to be doing so. Where he wanted to be flown was of course to his friend's boat, speeding somewhere towards us. Kevin circled around for a while until we eventually located it, and then Peter carefully strapped him back in the harness.

All the while we were acutely aware of the unspoken menace

behind the amiable, smiling countenance whilst he held his gun rock steady in the face of the gyration of the machine.

Half-way down to the boat, the balance of power began to shift; subtly at first, and then the further away he sank below us the more significant it became. Now he and the gun were swinging away wildly at the bottom of the winch cable, and we were sitting much more prettily at the top.

Kevin looked across at Peter, Peter at me, and finally I back at Kevin. Our bandit was now just a few feet from salvation, his friends on the boat reaching up to grab hold of him.

'Are we all agreed then?' asked Kevin in mid-hover, no word having passed between us.

'Agreed,' said Peter firmly.

'Agreed,' I reiterated.

'Then hold on,' said Kevin tersely, 'because this is where it all starts to get interesting.'

He suddenly thrust the helicopter forward, jerking our recent acquaintance right out of the clutches of his colleagues down below, and flew off at great speed. The winch cable trailed in our wake at an angle of forty-five degrees, our suspended passenger hanging on for dear life.

The look of surprise on his face was coupled with horror as he took in the realities of his predicament. All too soon this would be followed by anger at his new-found aggressors. Kevin was flying at top speed away from the boat, now disappearing from sight behind us as Peter and I hung over the side of the helicopter, reporting back what we could see.

'Shame he hasn't yet relinquished hold on his gun,' I observed with mild apprehension, 'and is now sort of pointing it up at us.'

'Isn't it just,' said Peter with commendable calm. 'By the way, Kevin, just to keep you informed . . . I think we're about to be shot at.'

'Are we indeed?' retorted Kevin grimly, as the ping of a bullet struck the side of the cockpit. 'Suppose we had better attend to that, then.' He put the helicopter into a steep dive, and my stomach rose up into my chest.

There was only ever going to be one winner, really, and as Paulo hit the water for the first time the gun came flying out of his hand. It disappeared beneath the waves just as he arose gasping and dripping from his first dousing.

'Winch him in,' came Kevin's voice over the intercom. 'All the way to the top – I can see the police boat, now, only about five miles away. Be there in a couple of minutes.'

We followed his directions and soon Paulo was lying in the back of the helicopter, where he lay still securely strapped into the harness, gasping and panting on his back.

'Mike,' called Kevin, gesturing towards the co-pilot's seat, 'take over for a moment, will you? Autopilot's on – just hold her straight and steady at three hundred feet like I showed you before. There's something I need to be doing, right now.'

I took my seat as directed while Kevin clambered past me into the rear compartment. I watched out of the corner of my eye as he grabbed hold of Paulo's collar and pulled him up to a sitting position where they stared at each other, face to face.

'I can cope,' said Kevin between gritted teeth, 'with having to fly out into the middle of the ocean to pick up pieces of garbage like you when your badly flown plane crashes into the sea. I can cope with the fact that in a country as poor as this you feel the need to smuggle drugs to make a tawdry living for you and your no doubt equally tawdry family. I can even cope with the fact that you are fat, and you are ugly, and so disgustingly smelly that I will have to scrub out my helicopter with bleach for a week to vanquish the taste of you in my nostrils.'

He started to unbuckle the harness. 'But what I cannot cope with,' he continued, lifting Paulo to his feet, 'is people who point guns at me, and start firing.'

And so saying he finally freed Paulo from the harness, waved him a gentle goodbye . . . and pushed him back over the side again.

* * *

They were a tough lot, some of these helicopter pilots. Most of them had flown several tours in Northern Ireland during the worst of the troubles and had nerves of steel beneath their outwardly congenial savoir faire.

I spent as much time as I could in the co-pilot's seat, flying virtually every day. Like the search and rescue squadrons back in the UK, all the crews I met were calm, efficient and supremely professional. Of all the time I spent in the RAF, these days of skimming the jungle beneath cloudless blue skies or flying round the perimeter of the sudden tropical storms were the happiest by far.

Belize was the only tour where I came to know some of the pilots as people, rather than generally intense individuals wandering around in glorified boilersuits, talking a language all of their own. There were one or two Tom Cruise (*Top Gun*) look-alikes with their fast cars and wrap-around shades, but these were the exception rather than the rule. It must have been one of this ilk, however, who was involved in the following, which may be an apocryphal story, but which I was assured was completely true.

A solo RAF pilot was flying his fast jet late one Friday afternoon in a deserted part of the country near a very long, very straight stretch of road. He knew that a friend of his was driving down the same length of road on his way home for the weekend, and would be in his very distinctive car. After circling the area a couple of times he duly spotted him, and decided to give him a surprise.

He flew his jet lower and lower along the valley, roaring up behind his friend, who was still totally unaware of his presence. As he flashed past, the bottom of the plane just scraped the roof of the car, both vehicles surviving intact, and he roared off into the sunset, performing a victory roll of salute.

Both the pilot and his friend thought this was a great joke, but unfortunately the authorities took a rather different view. Learning of this high risk escapade by some circuitous route, they tracked down the pilot by a process of elimination. He was court-martialled and unceremoniously dismissed from the air force in great disgrace.

The Saudi Arabian Air Force however, on hearing of this episode, were so impressed by the pilot's demonstration of flying expertise that they sought him out, and hired him on the spot.

There was the Harrier pilot who came out to join his girlfriend, an air traffic controller, for a four-month tour only to find disaster had apparently struck the day before his arrival. We had plastered both her legs and she lay prostrate on a stretcher by the runway, to be loaded up for departure back to the UK as soon as the plane was cleared for take off.

Geoff, her boyfriend, departed crestfallenly off to the mess, his dream of a foreign tour together in tatters. As soon as he was out of sight, we removed his girlfriend's plaster and sped her back to the bar, where she was sitting, innocence itself, when he walked in.

The look on his face was priceless.

Also present was the only pilot to have been shot down and captured during the Falklands war. He spoke little of his experience save for one late, late night in the bar, and all I can now remember is him recounting to us how he was looked after by a little old lady who kept bringing him cups of tea, and biscuits.

And then there was 'Scotty' Weir . . .

Scotty was a law unto himself. A huge Glaswegian helicopter pilot, he was rumoured to have been court-martialled for flying his machine down one of the main streets in Belfast and hovering outside the Ministry of Defence headquarters, to express his disgust at some administrative decision he was less than delighted about.

Such was his flying ability, however, he was apparently let off with a caution and allowed to remain in service provided he never undertook such a stunt again. Which he didn't . . .

Or at least, not for a couple of months or so.

The first time I met Scotty was the night of his arrival. We were in the bar late at night, and Scotty fancied a little entertainment.

'Who's for a trip into town?' he roared. 'I'd like to see a bit more of this hell-hole I've landed in.'

'We don't go into town at night,' I explained to him – town being Belize City, the capital of the country and some twenty miles down the road. 'It just isn't safe to travel in groups of less than ten or so, this time of the day.'

'Not safe?' he exclaimed. 'Well, we'll see about that, laddie.'

He turned and strode out of the bar, returning a couple of minutes later.

'You up for a trip then, doc?' he asked.

I looked up at him, towering more than half a foot above me.

'Love to, Scotty,' I said, 'but just the two of us . . .' I shrugged.

A huge grin split his craggy face, and he reached an arm up to the back of his neck, withdrawing an enormous hunting knife from a sheath he had concealed there. 'Och, you'll be safe with me, laddie, and my little friend here.'

And I was. Each time I was.

There was a small medical staff on the camp. The medical centre had just two doctors, myself and the army colonel, who was officially in charge. In addition there was a small but clean and highly efficient field hospital with a surgeon, an anaesthetist and a dentist, together with a dozen or so equally proficient back-up staff.

When I arrived the surgeon was Gavin, an army major (more about him later), but half-way through my tour he was replaced by Malcolm, a wonderful if slightly eccentric flight lieutenant in the air force. An excellent surgeon, and great company, Malcolm had difficulty sometimes with the practical aspects of life – in particular, working the CB radio with which all the army vehicles were equipped.

To drive from one side of the camp to the other you had to

cross the runway, calling the control tower for clearance as you approached. There was a clear, well-established procedure for this, which Malcolm was completely unable to grasp.

You would buzz the tower as you reached the track by the side of the airport, giving your name and rank, the call sign of the vehicle you were travelling in, and finally your position.

'I'm in the front, driving,' said Malcolm, perplexed, the first time he was preparing to cross.

The designated call sign of our medical vehicle was 4/4, which was the one thing Malcolm could generally manage to remember. His conversations with the tower were usually confined to a simple request.

'4/4 Malcolm here. Can I come across?'

The disturbing thing was, they always let him, he was so polite and disingenuous.

Malcolm was also an exceptionally talented and rumbustious rugby player, and took the opportunity of a game whenever his surgical duties would allow.

We were playing one afternoon when, after a seemingly innocuous tackle, an opposing forward collapsed in agony as a sickening crack split the air. Malcolm and I, being the only two doctors on the pitch, immediately rushed to his aid. The forward lay immobile on the ground, his face a ghastly ashen grey, his right foot bent at a seemingly impossible angle to the rest of his leg. Even I was feeling nauseous.

Malcolm, however, was cheerfully undeterred. He bent down, grasped the unfortunate man's foot and wrenched it back into position with a grating, crunching sound I can still recall to this day.

At this point I was looking urgently for somewhere to be discreetly sick, whilst twenty-seven other rugby players were busy fainting where they stood. Malcolm remained totally unfazed.

'Saves so much time later on the operating table,' he explained with a grin, 'if you attend to it straight away.' He stood up and stretched, his task complete. 'Right then,' he continued, as we waited for some poor soul to retrieve the ball from the alligator pool adjacent to the pitch, 'do you think we should restart with a scrum?'

As I stood with him later in the operating theatre, watching him expertly pin and plate the fracture, he gave me some lasting advice.

'Don't ever be afraid to intervene,' he said. 'You just have to seize the moment, and act.' His eyes twinkled. 'After all, they'll never know you haven't got a clue what you are doing, and somehow it always seems to work.'

Malcolm left the air force for civilian life a couple of years later and became, I believe, a highly respected Professor of Surgery in a major London teaching hospital, with his own Harley Street practice.

Sadly, despite on several occasions trying to arrange to meet up when we were both back in England, I never saw him again. He collapsed suddenly and died in his early forties, leaving the world of medicine a poorer place for his absence.

I was unable to attend his memorial service, but the memory of '4/4 Malcolm' lives on to this day.

Gavin, the army surgeon, had thick black glasses, a lugubrious face and a droll sense of humour.

Although not officially supposed to – I was expected to be available at all times for aero-medical evacuation emergencies – I would sometimes travel with the surgical team to the three outlying civilian hospitals where they held a clinic each week. The head of the RAF on the camp, Wing Commander Stevens, would turn a benign blind eye to these unofficial leaves of absence.

'If you don't tell me, I won't know,' he said drily. 'Just make sure you're on the end of a radio somewhere.'

The civilian hospitals were an eye-opener for one more used to the ordered, sterilised world I had previously worked in. In one small town to the north, for example, the operating theatre –

which was little more than a shack – actually had windows, but without any glass in them. Small boys would peer curiously through, commenting as we went along.

'What you doing there, then?' they might ask during an appendectomy, or 'Look at all the guts he's got.'

There was another hospital in the south which we would travel to on a Wednesday, operating in the morning, outpatients and preparing the following week's list in the afternoon. Here the patients lay on the floor, on dirty old blankets if they were lucky, bare boards if they were not.

The hospital could not afford a catering service, and patients had to rely on friends and family to bring food in for them. Gavin was a one man contraception service, undertaking eight or nine female sterilisations each morning.

It had been a long session. 'One more before lunch,' said Gavin, stretching and yawning. 'Can somebody go and get her, please?' There were no porters, and we had to fetch and carry each patient to and from theatre ourselves. Paul, the dentist, and the anaesthetist, Alex, were dispatched to the ward, returning ten minutes later with a woman in her late thirties lying on a trolley.

'This her?' asked Gavin, looking for an identifying label.

'Last one on the left, they said,' shrugged Paul. 'Last one on the left is what you've got.'

The operation complete, we decided to take a break and drive down to the river for lunch, and a beer. It was so peaceful there by the running water, listening to the birds singing, the crickets calling, dozing lazily in the midday sun . . .

'Bliss,' murmured Gavin sleepily. 'Absolute bliss. What more could a man ask?'

What more indeed.

But there was trouble in store, back at the hospital . . .

'You've sterilised the wrong patient,' said the theatre sister on our return.

'What!' screeched Gavin. 'What the . . . how could we have done?'

He glared across at Paul and Alex. 'Didn't you check who you were bringing, for Christ's sake?'

They looked at each other in bewilderment. 'Last patient on the left, we were told,' said Paul, a worried expression on his face, 'and last patient on the left is who we brought.'

But the last patient on the left had got up and gone off to the loo just a moment or two before Paul and Alex had walked in. There were no beds or cubicles demarcating where a patient should be, and no one who spoke English to put them right. When they had collected what they thought was the last woman on the left, she was in fact the last but one . . .

Gavin's face was ashen. It was his responsibility as the surgeon, and his alone, to ensure he was operating on the correct patient.

'They'll string me up and hang me out to dry,' he said faintly. 'Sorry for shouting, boys. It's my mistake, I have to take the blame.'

Surgical ruin was staring him in the face. With a heavy heart he sighed deeply and turned to the theatre sister. 'Is there a next of kin?' he asked wearily, rubbing his eyes with fatigue. 'I'd better go and talk to them, though goodness knows how I'm going to explain.'

The lady's husband was waiting outside the ward entrance. 'That's him,' motioned one of the nurses in Gavin's direction as we walked slowly into sight. He crossed to where Gavin had stopped, shaking perceptibly.

'Are you the surgeon?' asked the man.

'Yes,' Gavin nodded. 'I'm so sorry – '

But he got no further. 'Oh thank you, *thank* you,' said the man, and grabbing hold of Gavin's hand he pumped it up and down furiously, a huge beaming smile on his face. 'We both wanted her to be sterilised, the doctors said another pregnancy would kill her, but the hospital has so little money. They told us it would be another year, at least, before her turn would come. I can't thank you enough for fitting her in.'

* * *

Every officer on a six-month tour was allowed a two-week break. Some would have wives and girlfriends make the trip out to Belize, others choosing to travel back to the UK. In addition we would be given the odd long weekend to go and see parts of the country we had yet to visit. Four of us – two Harrier pilots, 'Boggo' and Steve, an air traffic controller, Chris, and I – made our plans. But it was not the delights of Belize, for us.

We chose to drive up to Mexico, instead.

The base had several cars available for hire, all of which were out on loan save for an old bus of a Cadillac, an automatic. I was in charge of supplying any medical equipment we might need in an emergency.

An English doctor in a foreign country often assumes an air of complete medical superiority over the local population. I did the same, packing enough medication and equipment to run a small general hospital throughout several major disasters.

'What's that?' asked Boggo, as I loaded the boot.

'Heroin,' I replied absently.

'In case we run out of money?' he asked, intrigued.

'No, to bribe the border guards with if they should find the cocaine,' I answered seriously. The trouble was he believed me, which says something about either my reputation or the gullibility of Harrier pilots.

We drove throughout the night, arriving at our destination in the late afternoon. Mexico has many sites of historical interest to explore . . . and we ignored them all, heading instead for Cancun, a large town in the east, and the night clubs, and the beach.

Our first night was spent on a 'Pirates' cruise to an island in the Gulf of Mexico, a quiet night out in the company of one's fellow tourists. To give you the general idea, drinks – Pina Coladas on the way out, Marguerita's and 'Slammers' on the return – were free throughout the excursion. Half an hour away from the shore, the maitre d' – a man so infuriatingly jolly we later felt compelled to debag him during the course of a limbo-dancing competition on the island – announced over the boat's Tannoy system that we were all invited to return to the bar for our second refreshment.

Which presented us with something of a problem, as we had already consumed five or six each. Somehow the evening began to deteriorate from that point onwards.

Our days were spent languishing on the beach, a glorious strip of golden sand and crystal clear waters. After two days it became common knowledge that I was a doctor, and English-speaking tourists would often wander over for advice. It had its advantages – primarily alcoholic in nature – and I was generally happy to oblige whilst still sufficiently sober to do so.

It was a dream holiday, the best I have yet had, but all too quickly the last day dawned. I awoke on the beach, recovering from the excesses of our previous evening and wondering where I had left my companions, and the hotel. As I waited for them to arrive from whatever dark hole they had finished up in for the night, I sat idly watching a grossly overweight middle-aged American venturing far out into the tumultuous surf between two ostentatiously sited red flags.

'Asking for trouble,' I murmured to myself, before dozing off back to sleep.

I am not normally so prescient, but trouble he got, and sooner than I had anticipated. I was woken by the sound of frantic shouts, and somehow I just knew what had happened. As I opened my eyes they were dragging his body head first out of the sea, his feet ploughing two deep furrows in the wet sand.

I watched from a safe distance, noticing with growing apprehension some of the gathering crowd glancing and pointing in my direction. Maybe they'll think I'm one of the pilots, or Chris, I thought, shrinking back down on my towel. Chris, incidentally, was the only man I ever met who, on arrival in a place like Cancun for a few days' hedonistic debauchery, could prepare by immediately unpacking his suitcase and ironing his silk pyjamas. Both pairs.

My attempts at anonymity might well have met with success had not my formerly mislaid companions arrived at precisely that moment, hailing me from the top of the beach with such witticisms as 'And where have you been all night?' and 'Break out the penicillin.'

It was inevitable. One of the crowd down by the sea broke away and ran across to where we were now all sitting, and stood panting in front of me.

'Are you the doctor?' he asked breathlessly.

I nodded.

'We need some help,' he said urgently.

I had no equipment or drugs, no stethoscope, and knew I would be of no assistance, but somehow I couldn't refuse.

'Please,' he begged. 'I think he's dying.'

I stood up reluctantly to follow him back to where the crowd was milling round the unfortunate bather. It reminded me of a fight in the junior school playground – the yard seems at first empty, and then suddenly all the schoolchildren are miraculously gathered around the protagonists, all jostling for position.

Chris thrust a gin and tonic into my hand.

'Drink,' he said simply. 'You'll be needing it.'

I approached the crowd, trying to clear my head, and then it came to me. This was the best – possibly the only – chance I had ever had to fulfil a lifelong ambition. I had once seen Marcus Welby do it in a television drama, and an eight-year-old's mind is so very impressionable.

I cleared my throat nervously and then announced in ringing tones;

'Make way. I'm a doctor.'

It was a supremely gratifying moment. The wall of bodies melted before me like the Red Sea, forming a corridor to where my patient-to-be lay in the inner circle. Then the wall reformed with me on the inside, and suddenly it wasn't gratifying at all.

The man was dead, I could see at a glance. He was lying flat on his back like a beached whale, eyes glazed, pupils already dilated, his mountainous stomach rising grotesquely into the air.

A coronary in the water, I thought immediately. No doubt dead as a doornail before they even got to him.

I looked around.

Every eye was upon me, every attention fixed on my presence, expectancy and anticipation in the air. I had arrived, the saviour. I was going to *do* something, I would revive him in a matter of moments. Thinking frantically, I glanced back down at the body. He was still dead, and going greyer by the second.

'Aren't you going to do anything, then?' said a young American man in an aggressive manner.

'Yes, come on,' said another. 'Happy enough to give advice when there's a drink in it for you, but when it comes to real medicine . . .'

It was completely hopeless. I was trapped, struck by the irony of having to try and resuscitate a pronouncedly dead stranger on a foreign beach some six thousand miles from home without so much as a stethoscope to aid me. There was no way out.

'Anyone here know anything about resuscitation?' I asked tersely.

The aggressive young American nodded curtly. 'Me,' he said. 'I've been on a course,' stressing the 'I've' as if he at least would know what he should be doing.

'Then why haven't you already started?' I wanted to say, but wisely thought the better of it.

I stood and considered the next step. There are two aspects to resuscitation – the mouth to mouth part, and the pushing on the chest bit. My corpse had a mouth full of sand, sea water . . . and vomit. My mind worked furiously.

'Big chap like this,' I said briskly, 'the heart massage is critical. I'll do that – you take the mouth to mouth. I'll tell you when to blow. OK with you?'

The American's jaw dropped, but he was as securely trapped as was I. He nodded his assent with evident distaste. For ten minutes we applied ourselves to the impossible task in my hands and his mouth, and all the time the crowd were gathering closer, the expectation tangibly growing.

It seemed nobody was aware that the man was very dead indeed, save for me. I wondered more and more how I was going to manage to break the news, becoming increasingly annoyed by the aggressive American's even more aggressive friend. 'Why don't you try This?' he would suggest, or 'Couldn't you try That?' and was there anything I wanted?

A mobile intensive care unit, I thought viciously, but kept quiet. Tension was mounting. Somehow I had to find a way out of this predicament, the sheer, mindless bloody stupidity of continuing to attempt to resuscitate a dead man for no other reason than I just didn't know how to stop.

And then it happened. That telling phrase, the apt response, that warm feeling you get when you say the right thing to the right person at the right time. The annoying friend said it once too often: 'Anything else you need?'

I stood up, and wiped my forehead. Everyone waited.

'Yes,' I said slowly. 'Anyone got a coffin?'

At the end of the fight, when the teacher arrives, the children all suddenly disappear, leaving the struggling combatants on their own. It was like that now.

What I had not known is that while we were occupied the dead man's wife had been found and had just arrived. She was standing right behind me. As she collapsed in hysterics and was led away, it all became very quiet. In a moment the beach was deserted. I was alone. In the midday sun the dead man and I stood and looked at each other, and I, at least, wondered what to do next.

In the end I collected some orange hotel towels that were lying nearby and carefully draped them over the body. And then, as the sun began to beat down in its fullest intensity, I left, looking back just once at the huge orange mound on the sand.

It would need to be a very big coffin, I thought.

9

A Little Trouble in
South America (Part 2)

RAF Belize, as we always referred to the base despite its preponderance of army personnel, was as previously stated some twenty miles from the capital of the country, Belize City.

As also mentioned the city was generally a no go area unless on official business during daylight hours; at night servicemen were only permitted to go there in large enough numbers to ensure their safety on the streets. But you cannot coop up an entire station of largely single – and, if married, almost always unaccompanied – young men for twenty-four hours a day.

People needed somewhere off camp to relax and have a few drinks in comparative safety, and this is where the Rose Garden – Rosie's, as it was universally known – came into its own. It was the only available drinking establishment between the camp and Belize City, situated about four miles from the gates of the base.

Its positioning was crucial to its success. It was close enough for people to reach – and, more importantly, stagger home from in the early hours of the morning – far enough from the city to be relatively trouble free, and just a sufficient distance from the camp for the hierarchy to turn a blind eye to precisely what went on there.

For the Rose Garden was more than just a meeting place for a few friends to have a quiet drink or two; more than just a safe haven from the hostile environment further down the road; and more than the pleasure of a leisurely evening stroll home in the

161

still, moonlit night to the tune of chirruping crickets and croaking frogs accompanying your journey with a melodious symphony all of their own.

Because the simple truth was . . . Rosie's was a brothel.

When you first arrived in Belize you stepped off the plane into an eight-hour jet lag. Landing at around four o'clock local time, you were all too well aware that it was heading for midnight, back home.

For the RAF in a mainly army environment, there would usually be only a couple of officers arriving on any one flight. That first evening was the unofficial initiation night – Flaming Drambuies, the true test of one's character, would follow later.

There was no standard ceremony, as such. The poor, exhausted, jet-lagged arrival was invited into the bar to be welcomed into their new environment, where all any of the old hands wanted to do was to see how long they would last. If you survived until eleven in the evening (about 7 a.m. the next day, back home in the UK) you were considered to be OK. Midnight, and you were a pretty good lad, and if you were to manage a visit to the Rose Garden . . .

As the evening wore on, the defining 'Are you a man or a mouse?' moment arrived.

'Anyone for Rosie's?' asked Alan, one of the communications officers, several hours into my first night. 'Neil, I know you will. Mike – would you care to join us?'

Mike did. I have no recollection of how we got there, this first time, but generally somebody present had access to a vehicle, and a driver, of some sort. It wasn't long before we realised that the one person who could be relied upon to be sober, ever present, and unable to argue with any senior officer who might be making totally unreasonable demands upon him was . . .

The duty ambulance driver.

He slept each night on the floor of the hospital reception area, to be immediately available whenever an emergency might arise. Emergency requirement to visit the Rose Garden whenever requested was not specifically mentioned in his terms of reference, but hey, he was Belizean, and a small tip or two was always a welcome addition to his meagre living.

Gavin, the army surgeon, had his own vehicle for much of the time. He could often be persuaded to drive it down if we caught him early enough in the evening for him still to be under the delusion that he would be sufficiently sober to drive it back again – up to a point.

That point, unfortunately, arrived the day we emerged after a longish refreshment session at around three in the morning to find the vehicle exactly where we had left it . . . but unfortunately minus all the wheels we had used to get it there.

'What is your favourite charity?' asked the Station Commander of him later that day.

'I beg your pardon, sir?' asked Gavin, taken aback.

'If you don't currently have one, adopt one in the next sixty seconds,' continued the Brigadier, 'and write me a cheque made out to them for £100 in memory of what used to be your vehicle. We will then consider the matter closed.'

A sensible man, the Station Commander, or so he seemed at the time. I just couldn't understand how he came to be in the services in the first place.

Standing outside Rosie's on that first night it seemed rather a pleasant spot – nice entrance, a few potted palm trees, doorman waiting to check you in . . . all very calm and relaxing.

Then you went inside.

Imagine if you can all the rugby players you have ever met scrummaging down at one and the same time with a beer in their hands, and you will have some idea of what Rosie's could be like. The place was heaving. We threaded our way across the floor to the bar, dodging the staggering and the lurching and stepping over the merely lying down and unconscious.

When finally we made it we stood with our backs to the counter, breathing deeply, surveying the scene of chaos and devastation that met our eyes in the semi-darkness.

The interior consisted of one enormous room with a bar running the entire length of one of the long walls. At one end a short flight of steps led down to a juke box and a tiny dance floor, and that was pretty much all there was save for a dozen or so bar stools and a few tables and chairs that were not yet broken beyond usage.

But it was surely only a matter of time.

'Nice place you've brought me to, Neil,' I observed.

'Ah, you just wait,' he grinned. 'Remember Bachman Turner Overdrive?'

'You ain't seen nothing yet,' I sang. (A classic from the sixties, for those too young to recall.)

'Precisely. Its full charms are yet to be revealed to you.'

As the hours slipped by I became cocooned in a state of suspended animation. By four in the morning much of the human debris had departed, and you could begin to get a grip on your surroundings.

I was sitting on a stool, leaning idly against the bar – a state I became remarkably familiar with over the next six months – when a small, dark-haired mustachioed chap to my right leaned across and tapped me on the shoulder.

'I hear you're the new doctor, then,' he slurred. News obviously travelled fast over here.

'I'm pretty sure I was when I arrived,' I admitted, 'but having been awake for the past thirty-six hours and drinking the last eight I'm not so sure any more.'

He waved a hand dismissively. 'Oh, you are all right. I've made it my business to know.' He tugged at my shirt and said in a stage whisper, 'We've got a proposition for you.'

'We?'

'Yes, we.'

He stood and leaned half way over the bar, beckoning to a

small plump man at the far end. 'Hey, Raouel. I think I've found just the man you've been looking for.'

Raouel walked across with nimble steps, and looked at me shrewdly through dark, heavy-lidded eyes. 'And who might that be?' he asked. 'The man from the immigration office with his head on a plate?'

'No,' said my companion. 'The new doctor.'

Raouel regarded me steadily. 'You?' he said after due consideration.

'Me,' I replied, ducking instinctively as a glass flew past my ear, a small fracas having broken out a little further down the bar involving three or four young soldiers and a chair. Raouel glanced across and sighed.

'Excuse me,' he said, 'I have a little work to attend to. You come back tomorrow?'

'Er . . . yes,' I agreed. 'When did you have in mind?'

'Corporal Richardson will bring you,' called Raouel over his shoulder. 'Won't you, Richie?'

'The pleasure will be all mine,' he confirmed, pointing to where Neil was gesticulating frantically by the door. 'I think your lift home is waiting, sir. I'll pick you up at two from the officers' mess tomorrow afternoon.'

The following morning I was taken on the 'Meet your elders and betters' introductory tour. The Station Commander, an army Brigadier, looked up without interest from some papers he was studying and said briefly, 'Good flight? Sergeant Jackson will show you back to your block,' before returning to the task in hand.

'And lovely to meet you too, sir,' I muttered under my breath.

The head of the smaller RAF contingent, Wing Commander Stevens, regarded me shrewdly. 'Ah, Sparrow,' he said. 'Your reputation precedes you. A message for you from the rest of the air force back in Britain – don't wind the army up. They have more men over here than we do, and higher ranking officers.'

'Thank you, sir,' I replied. 'I'll bear that in mind.'

'Be sure that you do,' he nodded, and I'm sure I heard him add softly as I left his office, 'Fat chance of that, I'll be bound.'

Next on my whistle stop tour was the hospital, where I was led through to the colonel in charge.

'Name?' he demanded, without looking up from his desk.

'Sparrow,' I answered mildly.

'Right,' he continued, still without raising his eyes from the notes in front of him, 'and your problem is?'

'Well,' I said, considering, 'I'm six thousand miles from home, a bit jet-lagged and I have a touch of a headache.'

He scrawled quickly on a prescription pad in front of him, tore the top sheet off and passed it to a young army private standing rigidly to attention next to him. 'Aspirin. Tell him to take two of them four times a day until his headache goes away. Next patient.'

Well, start as you mean to go on. I walked across to his desk, tore the prescription in half and dropped it on the table in front of him.

'I'm the new doctor,' I said softly, 'and if like me you had been taught to look at your patients every once in a while you might have spotted that, before now. Thanks for the advice, but with your permission I shall pass.'

And that was my introduction to Colonel Laverne, the start of a relationship which was given no chance to flourish. He went home on leave, two days later, never to return.

'Interesting consultation technique,' I remarked to Sergeant Jackson. 'Not one I've come across before.'

'Why do you think he's out here, sir,' responded Jackson darkly, 'begging the Colonel's pardon, of course. Not so many people to misdiagnose here as a normal base, if you'll excuse me saying so. Mind you, sir, the one before him was worse.'

How? I wondered quietly, but was never to find out.

From the hospital I was taken to the stores, the airfield, the helicopter squadron . . . and a whole load of other places I was to forget in an instant. I returned to the mess and sat with a beer, exhausted.

'Busy morning you've had, sir,' said Corporal Richardson in my ear, arriving true to his word on the stroke of two o'clock. 'And what a lot of nice new friends you seem to have made. Still, look on the bright side – made more of an impression in your first twenty-four hours here than your two predecessors in their entire stay. And all without trying, as well. Welcome to Belize, sir,' he added drily, 'and may your stay be a long and happy one.'

'Thank you, Corporal Richardson.'

'Richie, sir, it's easier. And . . . er . . . we usually refer to the junior officers as "Boss" or "Guv" – but if it's OK with you I guess we'll just call you Doc. Keeps it simple, that way, doesn't it, and then no one needs to bother with your name.'

'Suits me fine,' I agreed. 'I never was that much good at the protocol bit.'

Memories of 'Initial Officer Training' at RAF Cranwell came flooding back. 'If it moves, salute it,' the warrant officer in charge of us had barked fearsomely, 'and if it doesn't, paint it white.'

'Got a vehicle over at the stores,' pointed Richie, 'so as you seem to have the afternoon off . . .'

He drove me down to Rosie's, filling me in on some of the details.

'Always used to be looked after by the RAF doctor, the girls did, it was a traditional thing, but the last three before you . . .' He shook his head sadly. 'First one was some born-again religious freak, refused to go anywhere near the place. After him came Doc Watson, Amelia, but she only lasted a couple of weeks.'

'What happened to her, then?' I asked curiously.

'It was that time of the year,' he said with a grin. 'Those Nissen huts you sleep in, you have to shut the doors properly at night. Left them open, just the once she did, the one to the corridor and the one to her room on the latch in case anyone needed her in a hurry. Woke the entire camp up, screaming her head off in the early hours . . .' He bit his lip and started giggling.

'And?' I prompted him.

'Needed a pee in the middle of the night. Stepped out of bed without turning the light on . . . Land crabs,' he snorted, 'hundreds of the buggers attracted by the light in the corridor, scrambling over each other on the floor of her room. Had to sedate her for days . . .'

I shuddered. 'And after her?'

'Oh, Doc Peters, you met him briefly at the airfield. Said it was morally reprehensible and he wanted no part of it.'

'Well, I suppose you have to respect other people's principles and moral beliefs,' I said thoughtfully.

'Moral beliefs?' said Richie, raising an eyebrow sardonically. 'Moral beliefs – bollocks. Doc Peters moved one of the local women into his room, near as dammit, to do his washing and ironing and everything else that went with it.'

'OK,' I accepted, 'it may be a little morally ambivalent, but if he was single . . . I guess he wasn't single,' I finished weakly as Richie raised a contemptuous eyebrow.

'Wife and four kids, as far as I know,' he said disparagingly. 'Sanctimonious git, if you ask me. And then there were the snakes.'

'The snakes?' This was becoming more surreal by the moment.

'The snakes,' repeated Richie. 'In love with them, he was. Used to walk around with two baby coral snakes' (the most venomous creatures in the country) 'peeping out of his top pocket. Said it was to help people identify them more easily, but in all the time he was here the only person who ever got bitten was some poor bloody aircraftsman he handed one of them to so he could get a closer look. You've not that much of an act to follow, doc. Can't possibly be worse than any of them.'

'Thank you Richie,' I said sardonically, 'for your vote of confidence. It makes me feel so much more comfortable.'

By this stage we were drawing close to our destination. 'Before we go in, Richie,' I said, voicing a thought that had been on my mind for some time, 'why me, and not one of the army doctors? They must have the seniority, after all.'

'Well, you've met the Colonel,' he said, 'and there's not many sexually transmitted diseases they can cure with a couple of aspirin any more. And besides, there's the question of payment.'

'Payment?' I said, surprised. 'I hadn't thought . . .'

'Not yet, maybe,' grinned Richie. 'But it would have crossed your mind, sooner or later. I'll let Raouel explain.'

The bar was empty save for Raouel, who was totting up the previous night's takings. He motioned for us to take a seat.

'You want a beer or something?' he asked.

'What was that stuff I was drinking last night?' I asked Richie in an aside. 'Meths with a hint of paint stripper?'

'Two rum and Cokes, please, Raouel,' said Richie. 'I think I'll just leave you two together and take a little walk. OK with you, doc?'

'OK with me,' I agreed.

He departed in pursuit of his own affairs, nefarious or otherwise, as Raouel – surprisingly nimble for one of his circumference – vaulted the bar. There was no gap along its length. 'Is safer that way,' he said, noticing my glance, 'and stops the people trying to help themselves.'

He motioned to a table and drew up a couple of chairs. 'Please be sitting,' he said, gesturing. 'I tell you how I like to do things, and if you like too – is OK. You no like,' he shrugged, 'is still OK. We manage.'

It was all pretty simple, really. The army already had its own STD (Sexually Transmitted Diseases) clinic back at the camp, run by an army sergeant medic who was beyond being surprised. He operated with calm, unflappable efficiency, but was forbidden by his superiors to treat the girls at Rosie's.

With a little unofficial exchange of information, however, it was usually possible to figure out who had given what to whom, and how often, and treat appropriately. Raouel always stopped the girls from working if they had any symptoms, and would pay them a living wage until they had recovered, which surprised me at first.

'I stop their wages, they no tell me they diseased, more people catch from them, army stop people coming here . . . Is good business sense,' he explained, but I think he was a bit of a softie, at heart.

He wanted the girls to be checked at least monthly, and would supply one of the local nurses to help with all the routine swabs and checking. But most of all what he wanted was someone to see to them when they were roughed up – a not infrequent occurrence – and treat them when they were genuinely ill.

It was a delicate balancing act – the services turned a blind eye to what went on there as long as nobody overstepped the mark, and Raouel and the girls accepted behaviour up to a point, and occasionally beyond. It was a genuine symbiotic relationship, each needing the other to survive.

But never would you get either of them to admit it.

'So that OK with you?' asked Raouel, having explained what he wanted.

I nodded.

'Good,' he beamed, 'so now you be wanting to know about payment.'

'No, I don't need paying,' I said – yes, foolishly, I know. 'It's all part of the rich tapestry of life.'

'I say now you be wanting to know about payment,' he repeated firmly. 'That way you owe me nothing, and I owe you nothing either. Then we have no problems. You understand?'

I understood.

'Good,' he continued. 'Then you have two choices . . .'

He took me to meet the girls, after that. It may seem strange, referring to them as 'girls', but I never thought of them any other way, either then or now.

They ranged from the 'Wouldn't touch them with somebody

else's bargepole' variety to the indescribably beautiful, like Bernadette. Tall, elegant, with exquisitely chiselled features and long, beaded, dreadlocked hair, she was simply stunning, with a mischievous sense of humour, as well. Mostly, however, they were just young, pretty, illegal immigrants with other mouths to feed than just their own.

'So why do you do it?' I remember asking Monica, a delicate Mexican girl, one day.

She shrugged. 'It's a living,' she said resignedly. 'I have two children, no passport, and no man to take care of me. What do you suggest I do – run for President?'

What else indeed?

Over the coming months I came to know some of them well – no, not *that* well.

'You have the two choices,' Raouel had told me seriously. 'Free drink and entrance to the bar for your entire time here . . . or free women.'

I held his gaze for a moment. 'I think I'll take the free drink,' I said at last, and he grinned suddenly, his teeth a white flash in his dark face.

'Twelve years I have been here,' he said, 'and you the first one that wanted the drink.'

Now, I would like to think I have a smattering more morals than the average alley cat, but I have never considered myself a prude. Yet even I was taken aback by the attitude of many servicemen – yes, officers included – who attended the evening entertainment at the Rose Garden.

Apart from myself and the staff of the hospital, the only other person I can vouch for certain was never enticed around the back of the bar for 41 Belizean dollars worth of extra-curricular activity – 20 for the girl of your choice, 20 for Raouel, 1 for the sheets – was my regular companion, Neil, an avuncular, grey-haired photographic reconnaissance officer.

As well as radiating moral integrity, a beacon of respectability in a dissolute world, I had other more prosaic reasons for declining to partake. Treating venereal disease on a daily basis doesn't half make you disinclined to catch it.

And as for Neil . . . 'Oh, it's not the wife,' he admitted sheepishly one day, 'it's the mistress. I couldn't ever be unfaithful to her.'

Being the pillar of moral rectitude I so undoubtedly was, some of the other officers used to give me their money at an early stage in the evening, whilst common sense still prevailed. 'And don't, whatever you do, give it back to me,' they would stress firmly, 'no matter how drunk I get, no matter how much I beg you.'

'Mike, I need my $40 back,' they would plead in the early hours, 'I *need* it . . .'

At the end of my six-month tour I flew back to the UK and picked up an English newspaper at the airport. My blood ran cold as I read for the first time about this new killer disease called Aids, which neither I nor anyone else in Belize had yet encountered.

All the girls, all the servicemen, all those drunken liaisons for $41 in a cheap brothel back bedroom with nothing more to catch, so we all thought, than could be cured by a bit of penicillin . . .

How many people, I wondered . . .

The fateful evening, when it arrived, began quietly, like so many others before it.

Friday night, five o'clock, and it's happy hour in the officers' mess. Flying is finished for the week for the aircrew, save for those manning the helicopter on standby, and the base is winding down for the weekend. As the sun slips slowly towards the yardarm, everyone begins to gather in the bar.

We drink the local Belizean beer, kept cool in the mortuary behind the medical centre, gin with pink tonic (there are no labels on the soft drinks, so the tonic is dyed pink to distinguish it from the lemonade) and my favourite, Pina Colada, made with an unusual blend of constituents, but delicious all the same.

After the first hour or so it is time to move on to the Flaming Drambuies.

This was the second part of the initiation process for each new officer following the first evening's visit to Rosie's. The rules were simple, and one of the old hands would demonstrate just how it should be done. You had to fill a sherry glass right to the brim with Drambuie, set light to it, and as soon as you saw the bluey flame skimming the surface you had to drink it as fast as you could. Couldn't be easier. Except that the longer you leave it, the hotter it gets.

Which is where the man with the bucket of water comes in.

All novices to the game, particularly those with significant facial hair, were warned that their face might catch alight. 'But no one has ever needed plastic surgery yet,' they would be reassured. 'And anyway, if that should happen the water puts it out very quickly.'

You've probably guessed by now. The new arrival drinks the Flaming Drambuie, everyone holds their breath . . . and the man with the bucket of water tips it over their head, no matter what else is happening. And once the first bucket of water has been thrown . . .

The officers' mess was shared by both army and RAF personnel. The bar staff, however, were always young airmen, which sometimes created a little tension between the two services. The majority of all officers treated them with respect, but there was a hard core of mostly army staff who were unpleasantly rude, which of course made the RAF even more protective.

But worse even than that was one particular officer, an army major, a tall, heavily built, ruddy-faced man who was over-friendly, over-polite . . .

'Nice, that Major Robinson,' said young Tom one day, as he was cleaning some glasses. 'Always buying the boys a drink or two down at Rosie's.'

Neil and I exchanged a glance. 'Just you be careful of him,

Tom,' I warned. 'I'd be happier if he was buying drinks for the girls.'

'You mean . . . ?' asked Tom, startled. 'Surely not, the Major's not like that. Just being friendly, he is.'

'Maybe so. But just be careful,' I repeated, 'that's all.'

Major Robinson and I had disliked each other from the start. On this particular evening he was standing on his own next to the door at the far end of the bar, well away from the flying buckets of water amongst the juvenile RAF contingent.

You could see how it happened. Two of the Harrier pilots, Boggo and Jonesy, slipped out of a side door, giggling like schoolchildren. A minute later I crossed the bar on my way to the loo and went out of the door next to where Robinson was still standing. A minute after that, Boggo and Jonesy entered the same doorway, threw two buckets of water over the back of the totally unsuspecting Major and fled back out of the door before he had time to turn round from his soaking and espy the culprits.

I then re-entered the bar a few seconds later, like an immaculately timed entrance in a Brian Rix farce, unaware of what had happened.

But not for long.

'You!' exploded Robinson as he turned and saw me standing in front of him. 'How dare you . . .'

He flashed out an arm and the back of his hand caught my cheek, although whether he meant it or not I am uncertain.

But it stung.

The next minute was rather a blur, and then I became aware of a tug on my shoulder. 'Let him go, Mike, for goodness sake. What the hell do you think you are doing?'

The red mist parted. Robinson was backed against the corner of the bar, my hand around his throat, his face becoming an interesting shade of red.

'It wasn't me,' I repeated between gritted teeth as I reluctantly relinquished my grip, 'and you owe me an apology.'

'Apologise?' he spat out. 'To you? It doesn't matter if it was you or one of your pathetically childish friends over there. You're all the same, little boys trying to do the job of grown men. You're not even worthy of my contempt.'

He stood back, straightened his tie and his cuffs, and walked out of the bar to snorts of derision.

'End of round one,' said Boggo cheerily, clapping me on the shoulder. 'Care for a drink?'

And there it might all have ended.

But it didn't.

The evening wore on as Friday evenings usually did, out there.

A few fell inevitably by the wayside, but sometime beyond midnight the still partying hardy perennials made our way past Jimmy, the doorman, into the sweating, heaving morass of humanity that was Rosie's at this early hour of a Saturday morning.

Charley, the barman, waved a bottle at us as we squeezed our way through to the bar, and I nodded gratefully. 'I'll put your name on it,' he grinned, reaching behind him for the Coke.

By three in the morning only Neil and myself remained of our original party. Rosie's was still packed, but even we were flagging.

'Time to go?' mouthed Neil, tapping his watch.

'Yes,' I nodded, mouthing back. 'Good idea.'

We walked across to the bar to wave goodbye to Charley, and there he was. Major Robinson, sitting on a stool up at the bar, drink in his hand. I couldn't help myself. I took a step towards him.

'No,' groaned Neil beside me. 'Let's go home, Mike, please just let's go home.'

'I'll only be a moment,' I promised. 'I just want a little chat.'

Robinson looked up disdainfully as I approached.

'Major Robinson,' I said with over-emphasised politeness. 'Just thought I would give you another chance to apologise.'

'You?' he slurred. 'Apologise to you? Whatever makes you think

175

I would want to do that? You're not worth any apology of mine.' And so saying he looked away again, resting his elbows on the bar.

I half-turned, clenching my fist. 'Walk away, Mike,' a voice was saying in my head, 'just walk away and forget it.' And I almost did.

'Oh, no,' moaned Neil again, 'oh please, no,' as I turned once more, called, 'Hey, Robinson,' and, as he glanced up swung the most beautiful left hook imaginable on to the point of his chin. A look of blank astonishment flashed across his face, and then he toppled slowly backwards off his stool, towards the floor.

That was bad enough in itself, but worse was to follow.

At this hour of the morning not everybody present was sober, or indeed conscious. In dissolute corners and dark holes around the place were servicemen crashed out in various states of disarray, and lined up against the bar in a neat row behind the now falling Major Robinson were six comatose soldiers on bar stools, fast asleep on the counter.

As he fell backwards on to the first of these, so he in turn toppled over too, and on to the next, like a row of dominoes . . .

'Oh shit,' said Neil's voice faintly behind me.

For the first time in our numerous visits the place became eerily quiet, everyone standing motionless, watching the almost comically slapstick pageant unfold. As the sixth soldier crashed to the floor, the mood began to turn ugly.

'Mike,' said Neil urgently, 'have you noticed that we are the only two RAF officers in the bar amongst a hell of a lot of very drunk soldiers, seven of whom you've just laid out on the floor?'

I was noticing fast. Goodness knows what might have happened – a scuffle had already broken out to our right, and several people were looking towards us with mutinous glances. We backed up against the bar, thinking furiously.

'Hey, doc,' called a voice behind us. Charley was beckoning furiously. 'This way, quick.'

Neil and I glanced at each other and nodded a rapid agreement. We dived over the bar, ducking down behind its sturdy protection as the first glass flew through the air and smashed against a mirror above our heads. Keeping low we followed Charley out through a store room, through the girls' working rooms and out through a back door into the fresh air, and the exhilaration of freedom.

'I can't get you out of this one,' said the Wing Commander, shaking his head sadly as I stood in his office two mornings later. 'Major Robinson has made a formal complaint. For God's sake, Mike, what on earth did you think you were doing? I thought you might have learned your lesson after last time.'

The last time he was referring to was an evening I spent in the bar in the company of the Grenadier Guards, of which the less said the better. Suffice to say that Scotty Weir was woken from his slumbers to come and rescue me from a fate worse than death, which he did by the simple expedient of picking me up and carrying me away over his shoulder until I promised not to go back again.

The next morning I crept in early and left a short message on the bar shutter. 'Flight Lieutenant Sparrow would like to apologise to everybody . . .'

'But no,' he sighed. 'I'm afraid it's out of my hands now. The Brigadier wants to see you.'

The Brigadier saw me, and he was not a happy man. By the time he had finished with me, however, he was an awful lot happier than I was.

'Hitting a senior officer is a court-martial offence,' he said coldly. 'I am sure you are aware of that.'

'I am, sir,' I replied quietly, 'but I would just like to say – '

The look on his face brought me to an abrupt halt. 'You can save what you have to say for the VJ,' he said, the words striking a chill to my heart. 'He's due out here in two weeks' time.'

VJ. The Visiting Judge, who travelled out to the foreign bases to hear all the more serious disciplinary cases. Had he not been due on a routine visit in so short a time I would almost certainly have been sent back to the UK for disposal there. But out here, in army territory . . . ?

This was getting serious.

I had no defence. I was guilty as charged, and I had the sneaking feeling that being drunk and starting a riot in a brothel were unlikely to be considered mitigating circumstances.

A court martial, and the inevitable conclusion, would mean the end of my career. Discharged without honour, only half-way through my vocational training, and a mountain to climb to find anyone to accept me for the rest of it.

This time, I had finally done it.

But worse, if that were possible, was to follow.

'In the meantime,' continued the Brigadier, 'you are strictly confined to camp. In addition, as you have demonstrated so clearly that you obviously cannot be trusted to behave in the manner your status as an officer demands of you after you have had a drink, you are henceforth banned from the bar.'

My misery was complete.

As luck would have it Dave Wingate, the RAF administrative officer, was due a spell of leave back in the UK. He was on a three-year tour in Belize with his wife and two children, and as such had his own bungalow within the confines of the camp.

'Could do with a house-sitter,' he said thoughtfully, jingling the keys in front of me. 'Can you think of anyone who might be available?'

'Thanks,' I said, holding out my hand.

'And I've stocked up with beers and the odd bottle of gin,' continued Dave, smiling. 'After all, he didn't say you couldn't drink, did he? Just that you couldn't drink in the bar.'

The next two weeks were a nightmare. Some days seemed

interminable, the hours dragging tortuously by, while others just flew past as if determined to speed me towards my doom as fast as they possibly could.

Opinions in the camp were divided. Although there were some who felt I was receiving my just deserts, and not a moment too soon, there was less general army disapproval than I had expected. Major Robinson was not a universally popular man.

'Almost wish I'd done it myself,' confided one captain with a wistful look in his eye. 'Not so keen on the court martial, of course, but hey – what a way to go . . .'

My friends were wonderful, to a man.

I had retired disconsolately to Dave and Carol's bungalow after dinner on the first night of my exile, resigned to a solitary evening watching the TV. Five minutes later there was a knock on the door, and when I opened it there stood Neil, Kevin, Chris and Jonesy with a crate of beer and a bottle of gin.

'Well, if you cannot go to the bar,' explained Neil solemnly, 'we thought that maybe we had better bring the bar round to you, instead.'

Night after night they came round to see me, but as the fateful day approached even their mood became progressively sombre.

'So what will you do, Mike?' asked Neil late one evening as he and I sat alone together, sharing a last drink.

To my horror I could feel a lump developing in my throat, and turned hurriedly away.

'I don't know,' I said simply. 'I just don't know.'

The day of the VJ's arrival finally dawned.

Planes flew in from the UK once a fortnight, bringing visitors, supplies, new arrivals and those returning from leave. I drove down to the airstrip to collect Dave, Carol and their children.

'House still in one piece then?' he asked, adding shrewdly, 'You still in one piece, too?'

'I've been well looked after,' I said, and grinned. 'The

179

condemned man has been eating rather a lot of hearty breakfasts, figuratively speaking.'

'I sat next to the VJ on the plane,' said Dave quietly, as we drove back towards the camp. 'His name's Crawford. He was asking about you.'

'And?'

'His hands are tied, Mike. No one really wants to hang you out to dry, but you can't set a precedent, especially out here – it's too isolated. Hitting a senior officer only ever results in one decision – even if the officer in this case was only Robinson. But Crawford is a smart guy, got his head well and truly screwed on. "It isn't going to be a witch hunt," he told me, "despite what some of the more senior army officers would like to see. But due legal process must be adhered to, and justice – no matter how pedantic it may be – has to be seen to be done."'

'Meaning he's going to have to make an example of me, whether he wants to or not?' I said bitterly.

'Meaning he's got a job to do. "So what do you call justice?" I asked him, and for what it's worth, he winked at me. "Justice," he said, "is like beauty. It's in the eye of the beholder."'

We sat in silence for the rest of the journey, and I dropped them off at their bungalow.

'Thanks for the lift, Mike,' said Dave, 'and now just promise me one thing. Whatever you do, please, *please* – don't get into any more trouble tonight.'

There was a special dinner on in the mess.

A group of visiting dignitaries had arrived on the same plane as Dave and the VJ, and a lavish banquet had been laid on in their honour. Even I had to eat, but with dinner came wine, and plenty of it. It would have been churlish not to have partaken.

As the evening progressed, a devil-may-care attitude began to creep steadily over me. Eat, drink, and be merry, for tomorrow . . .

I tried to suppress the thought.

The party moved on to the bar, spilling over into the open-air section covered by the atap, just outside. I made my way reluctantly back to my room to decide how I was going to approach the coming ordeal, but just as I reached the accommodation block I heard footsteps rushing up behind me.

'Of course, you might be banned from the bar,' said Neil thoughtfully as I turned to face him, 'but the path bordering the atap can't be included as part of the bar, now can it, strictly speaking?'

'I think you might have a point there,' I said slowly, considering.

'And anyway,' continued Neil brightly, 'it's open to interpretation, and there's only one way to find out. Come and have a drink, Mike, and to hell with the lot of them.'

I stood for a while on the path outside the bar while they brought me out drinks, and then I stood under the atap while they brought me out some more. I was just about to throw caution to the winds when I saw the Wing Commander bearing down upon me, and froze upon the spot.

'Relax, Mike,' he said, catching the expression on my face. 'It's an air force do tonight. Twenty-four hour amnesty granted, on my authority.' He put an arm around my shoulders and led me towards the bar. 'And besides, Susie' (his wife) 'sent me out to get you. She'd like to buy you a pint.'

Susie, a tanned, sultry blonde with a husky voice, was talking to an engineering officer, another Neil – Neil II as we called him – as we approached.

'. . . so if you show me your white bits,' she was promising, 'then I'll show you mine.'

'Really?' said Neil II, uncertain. 'Here? In the bar?'

'Right here,' purred Susie. 'But you first.'

Neil considered carefully for a moment, and then went for it. Undoing his flies, he dropped his trousers to the floor and revealed a pair of lily-white buttocks to general cheers all around. With a self-conscious grin on his face he bent down and pulled them up again, waved in good-natured acknowledgement, and turned back to Susie expectantly.

'You promised,' he said. 'We all heard you.'

'Yes, I did, didn't I?' agreed Susie, smiling broadly. 'Well then, here goes . . .'

She held up her left hand and slowly, seductively, slid her wedding ring down her finger. A thin circle of white glowed luminously in the soft lighting of the bar. 'There,' she said, looking Neil II straight in the eye, 'that's the only white bit I have left . . .'

The evening progressed, and deteriorated.

At one in the morning there were still quite a few of us left. Susie had departed with a squeeze of my hand and a nod in the direction of her husband.

'Best of luck for tomorrow, Mike. And don't worry about him – he says you may have given him more headaches than any other doctor we've ever had but you're actually a damn sight more efficient than any of them. He'll put in a good word for you, I know he will.'

The bar was closing, at last.

'Looks like it's Rosie's, then,' said Jonesy. 'See you in the morning, Mike.'

'So you'd leave me here then, would you?' I sighed. 'On my last night of gainful employment, deserted by my friends, cast adrift into an ocean of uncertainty . . .'

'No,' said Jonesy firmly. 'You can't.'

'No,' echoed Neil, more firmly still. 'It would be suicidal.'

'And yet,' considered Neil II, 'come to think of it, what more can they do to you? You might as well go out with a bang, mightn't you?'

He looked around appealingly to the others, and slowly, after a few moments' thought, heads began nodding.

'Indeed I might,' I agreed.

Rosie's, as ever, was packed.

'Watcha, doc,' greeted Jimmy at the door. 'Back where you belong.'

'For the last time, Jimmy,' I answered. 'You going to let us in?'

He grinned, big white teeth flashing in the darkness. It was the last time I ever saw him – a week later he was murdered, a shotgun blast to the head, another casualty of the lawlessness of the place we mostly managed to avoid.

Charley, at the bar as ever, had already poured the drinks by the time we had side-stepped our way through the crowd.

'Figured you'd be in,' he chuckled. 'News travels fast around here. Raouel says everything's on the house – including Bernadette, if you're interested.'

The cares of the world began to slip from my shoulders.

'To your court martial,' said Jonesy, raising his glass and downing his drink in one. 'Who wants to stay in the air force for ever, anyway?'

'To my court martial,' I acknowledged, and we all raised our glasses in salute.

The drinks flowed freely, Charley's measures becoming larger by the round. After half an hour or so I had long forgotten the fact that Rosie's was the last place on earth I should be at such a time. Bernadette, looking even more stunning than ever in a simple white dress, was in mourning. She had fallen in love with Scotty, who was now back in the UK, and was consoling herself by awarding marks out of ten for all the men in the bar.

At two thirty in the morning I was sitting reflecting that life was not so bad after all. Tomorrow was just a minor blip on the horizon, there were other jobs, more lucrative careers . . . Maybe this would be my launching pad for some better, brighter future, the tide which taken at the flood would . . . would . . . well, would do whatever it was Shakespeare had said it would.

And then I saw him.

For a moment the crowds had parted, and there was Robinson, the man responsible for my current plight, sitting at a table amongst a group of young soldiers and airmen.

There was Robinson, laughing, drinking, playfully ruffling the hair of the soldier next to him. There was Robinson, enjoying himself without a care in the world, while I . . .

I watched him intently for a few moments, unable to avert my eyes, and then the gap through which I was watching closed up as quickly as it had opened. I sat, lost in thought, until Neil tapped me on the shoulder, a fresh drink in his hand.

'One for the road, Mike? And then we'd best be getting you home.' He peered closer. 'You all right, Mike? Seen a ghost or something?'

My court martial was set for the following afternoon.

I made breakfast, to everyone's surprise, and sat idly listening to the conversation around me.

'Bit of trouble down at Rosie's last night, then,' said Mark, one of the RAF regiment officers. 'And for once Sparrow doesn't appear to have been part of it,' grinning in my direction.

'So what's that then?' I asked without much interest. There was always a bit of trouble down at Rosie's, one way or another. A little more was of no consequence to me.

'Not sure of the details,' continued Mark, wrinkling his nose in disgust as he critically viewed the contents of his plate. 'What is *that*, for goodness sake? Have they forgotten how to cook an egg in this place?'

He took a tentative bite, and shrugged. 'Could be worse, I suppose. Some young airman or other,' another mouthful, 'has made a complaint. MPs' (Military Police) 'are buzzing about all over the place looking for anyone who was there, but they're not saying why. Of course,' he added, raising an amused eyebrow, 'it wouldn't be of any interest to you, being banned from the place, because you wouldn't have been there last night in any case, would you?'

I thought back to the previous night, much of which had passed in a blur. Jimmy, Charley, too many rum and Cokes . . . Bernadette, Neil and Jonesy . . . It hit me like a thunderbolt. Robinson. Robinson had been there. Oh my God, what had I gone and done this time?

And then I remembered . . .

The VJ, Colonel Crawford, stood up to greet me as I entered the room.

'Well, young Sparrow,' he said not unkindly, 'I've been hearing rather a lot about you from a variety of sources.' He waved towards an armchair by the wall. 'Take a seat. I've been looking forward to this.'

I sat as directed, my heart racing as he perched on the end of his desk.

'So, why don't you give me your account of your little contretemps with authority in the shape of Major Robinson,' he continued, and I swear there was a glint of amusement in his eye. 'And . . . um . . . we'll keep this off the record, for now, if that's OK with you.'

So we sat, he and I, just the two of us, as I ran through my tale. It was now midday, and my court martial was due to begin in two hours' time. When I got to the point where I described Robinson falling backwards off his stool and starting the domino effect down the length of the bar I could see Crawford biting his lip before turning away in an effort not to let me see him smiling.

'Well, that's it, sir,' I said, as I reached the end. 'The whole sorry story, I'm afraid. I'd like to say I regret it, but in truth I don't at all.' He turned back to look at me, a questioning expression on his face. 'Sir,' I continued, 'I know the rules as well as anyone else. I know what you have to do.'

'Do you indeed?' He stood up and walked across to the window, beckoning me over. 'See that room over there?'

I nodded, wondering what was to come next.

'Well, that is where you and I and a few other people are due to meet in a more official capacity in a couple of hours' time,' he said. 'And that is where under ordinary circumstances I would listen to what everybody has to say, and then usher you gently out of the country and service life, returning you back to an uncertain future in the civilian world. But these are not ordinary times, are they, and we have a bit of a problem.'

He turned round to face me again. 'Tell me, young man – was it a *very* good punch?'

I looked him squarely in the eyes. 'It was a beauty, sir,' I said proudly.

'I would have loved,' he sighed wistfully, 'to have been there to see it. Now,' he added, suddenly businesslike, motioning back towards the chair, 'you'd better sit down again and tell me what happened last night.'

'It's an unusual situation,' he said slowly as I finished, waiting to see what he was going to do. 'To be honest with you, I can't abide officers like Major Robinson, and perhaps more importantly for us both, neither can the army. And think of the publicity . . .'

He shuddered, considering the prospect.

'You are probably there ahead of me,' he resumed. 'I spoke to Major Robinson this morning, and no . . .' as I looked up, questioning, 'he doesn't know you are here now. He made my skin crawl, to be honest, and he still thinks he is to be the star witness in your thoroughly deserved comeuppance this afternoon. It's ironic, isn't it? I've never come across it before, he's the only witness against you, and you . . .'

He paused, and gazed across at me as if deciding how to proceed.

'You know what I'd be doing right now, if you were me and I was you?' he said unexpectedly.

We were reaching the critical point of our conversation. He was giving me a chance, and I had to get it right.

'I guess you would be offering me a deal, sir,' I said with a deep breath, taking my life in my hands.

He exhaled slowly. 'So I would, young man, so I would. Now, what precisely do you think it would be that I might have in mind?'

The crowds had parted, and Robinson was fully in my sight. I had been unable to remember, at first, and then just when I needed it most the entire episode came flooding back into my mind.

Robinson had reached across to the young soldier next to him, the same one whose hair he had earlier been playfully ruffling, and put his hand firmly behind his neck. As I watched, scarcely believing what I was seeing, he had pulled the soldier towards him and kissed him fully, slowly and lingeringly on the lips.

In all the bar, amongst all the people who were there, singing and drinking and revelling in the early hours, only one man had witnessed the entire event.

The man who was due to be court-martialled, the next day, for knocking him out.

We negotiated, Colonel Crawford and I.

The scandal of the case, had it come to court in that political era, would have been appalling. A respected army major French kissing a young private in a brothel in a country where the future of the armed services was already in debate . . . it was dynamite in the making. If the *Sun*, or the *News of the World* were to get hold of it . . .

It didn't bear thinking about.

'An amnesty,' I suggested. 'No court martial, no return to England before the predetermined end of my tour, and most importantly of all, a rescinding of my confinement to camp, and my ban from the bar. On the understanding,' I added hastily, 'that I more or less behave myself for the rest of my time here – meaning no hitting senior officers again, that sort of thing.'

'And in return?' asked the Colonel quietly.

'My silence,' I said simply. 'No mention of this conversation, no going to the newspapers, no referring to this whole episode in any capacity until, say, you and I have each been a civilian for at least ten years.'

Major Robinson, I understand, was offered a quiet resignation, without either disgrace or his pension. The young private was apparently offered an immediate posting, and promotion, as long as he withdrew the charges.

Both accepted.

And me?

I was offered back my future.

'It's a deal,' said Colonel Crawford with a smile, and shook me firmly by my hand.

10

Death in Strange Places

It's a funny thing, death, when you come to think of it. Along with our birth it's the only experience in life we all share, yet we recall nothing of either.

We may witness other births, with varying degrees of emotion, but we shy away from death as much as we are able. As a child, our grandparents may die but that is OK – they're old, and they're supposed to, it's what grandparents are for once they've stopped buying us Easter eggs and Christmas presents.

It's just part of the natural progression – or regression – of life. Isn't it?

But unlike our predecessors, few of us see death in all its tragic reality. It serves as a reminder of our own mortality, the ultimate memo on our checklist for life. So we are unused to it, unprepared for it, unwilling to contemplate the stark realities without the support of devout religious beliefs. One day it really will end, and we will be gone.

However to those of us in the medical profession, amongst others, death is just another part of life, and we deal with it accordingly. It may be why our attitude is slightly different . . .

When I became a medical student I had never seen a dead body, and scarcely knew anyone who had. It was one of those enigmas of life that seemed entirely irrelevant to me – I was not about to die, so why should I be unduly concerned about those who already had?

The medical school had a sympathetic, understanding approach to the delicate natures of innocents such as myself and my fellow students. After the gentle introductory lectures of the first day, and the raucously alcoholic events of the subsequent first night, they led us – green at the gills as we were – to the top floor of the medical school and propelled us gently into the anatomy room.

Mindful of our innocence, and having considered all the options, they adopted a variation on the desensitisation approach. You may not know the theory behind this, so let me explain.

Imagine you have a phobia about spiders, and run screaming each time you should see one. You begin your therapy by sitting in a quiet room, a spider-free zone, with a psychotherapist as your only companion.

After some relaxation therapy, with soothing music and perhaps a sherry or two, you begin talking in a roundabout way of the dreaded arachnids. The conversation drifts away each time you become tense, shifting on to some altogether less stressful subject matter – meeting the in-laws for the first time, perhaps, or explaining to your father how you managed to put such a very large dent in his brand new car when he had expressly forbidden you to drive it until after you had had your first lesson. As your breathing rate settles the conversation gradually returns to the subject in hand.

Soon you can talk about spiders like an enthusiast. Moving on you progress in leisurely fashion to pictures of spiders, films of spiders, and then corpses of spiders and their families. You begin to empathise with all those little problems in their lives – how best to spin that next web, can you make that one fly last until tomorrow's breakfast, what are you to do about that family of growing starlings looking ever more hungrily at you with each passing day?

Pretty soon they become your friends. Little spiders, big spiders, furry ones and scaly ones, you begin to love them, nurture them, long to have them crawling over your body in great profusion. Then you begin to fantasise about them . . . but only if you have a really good psychotherapist.

So we trailed dutifully into the anatomy room, eagerly anticipating the prerequisite couple of sherries before our ordeal. There before us was the carefully prepared dissection room with twelve naked dead bodies laid out on slabs. I think this comes under the category 'Accelerated Desensitisation'.

Three students fainted – interestingly all men, although one had previously collapsed in the corridor before going in and I'm fairly sure the corpses were not entirely responsible. One was sick in the corner, and another more indiscreetly over the senior anatomist's white coat. But the reaction I remember most vividly was that of a small Welsh girl who pulled a railway timetable from her coat pocket and looked up the first available train home.

Those of us later blessed were in due course invited into the inner sanctum. If you have ever watched the film *Coma*, you may have an inkling of what we saw. In the preparation room the bodies were removed from their various packaging – I once saw one covered from head to toe in twenty first birthday paper, a pink bow tied beautifully around her midriff.

Finally, if you had survived all the tests along the way, you passed through into the room that *really* mattered. In this most surreal of rooms, body upon body hung suspended upside-down from a row of butcher's hooks on an electrically controlled conveyor belt. At a given signal each would move silently forward to be dipped head first into a vat of formalin and rest there, greedily absorbing the stringent preservative fluid.

The memory is etched impermeably on my brain, along with the sight of my very first full bedpan and the look on the face of the senior biochemist when we inadvertently encountered him in the snooker room late one night in a position I would have previously thought anatomically impossible with a leading light of the Christian Union, who was apparently too busy to be immediately aware of our presence.

Death should not be funny, but sometimes it just is. People, sadly, do not all peacefully pass away in their sleep in gentle relaxed circumstances. They drop down all over the place. Fields, cars, planes – hospital, of course, goes without saying – trains, buses, and once – honestly – I had a patient drop dead in a mortuary whilst they were viewing their recently departed, who had, if I remember rightly, succumbed in a church whilst at a funeral!

Dying in the bathroom is commonest when at home and there is, I have to say, nothing so undignified as departing one's mortal coil whilst seated upon the lavatory. The patient – or ex-patient, to be more precise – is beyond caring, but I always feel so sorry for the relatives.

I was once summoned to the home of an elderly lady whose husband had died in just such a manner.

'He was such a dignified man,' she told me sadly. 'He would have hated it so. I know I don't know you, doctor,' (I was doing a locum at the time) 'but I wonder . . . I would be so pleased . . . would you . . . I've cleaned him up, you see, and put on some clean clothes but he is too heavy for me . . . I don't want anyone to know. Would you mind?'

'Of course not,' I replied, with gentle understanding and the knowledge that by the end of the day I would be back home in my practice over two hundred miles away. 'I would be glad to help.'

So I carried the late Mr Blenkinsop out of the toilet, down the hall, up the stairs – and I can tell you, he was getting heavy by now (I have resisted the temptation to call him a dead weight for the sake of a cheap laugh) – and laid him upon his bed. I staggered back downstairs, sweating slightly, and Mrs B followed a few moments later.

'I'm so grateful to you, doctor,' she said, 'and all his friends can come and see him now.' She leant forward confidentially. 'And you know what, doctor, he looked so worried when I found him. I knew what he was thinking – we've been married sixty years, you know, and I just knew how he would feel.'

She looked around with a sort of pantomime 'he's behind you' air, and laid her hand on my knee. 'And when I just left him, I swear he was smiling. He's happy now, I'm sure of it, and so am I.'

I left her then, mildly bemused. Her husband dies unexpectedly after sixty years of what seemed to be a blissfully happy marriage, and far from being distraught she was just happy that, to the outside world, he had died with his trousers on. Which, of course, not everybody does . . .

I was once called by a friend in a state of extreme panic. She had been having a long-standing affair with a very large, very rich and no longer very young colonial businessman, who from the look of him – ruddy face, huge belly and a tendency to turn blue round the gills when stepping up a kerb – looked ready to go at any minute.

I used to joke with her that it was bound to happen at the most inopportune of moments, to which she would regularly reply that inopportune moments were few and far between these days and never lasted long enough for him to die during. But the inevitable eventually occurred, and one day he did.

'It's happened,' she hissed over the phone, 'and it's your fault.'

'What has?' I wondered. 'And why?'

'Because you kept saying it would, you know what has happened and please will you bloody well come and get me out of this mess before his wife comes back and finds us here together.'

She explained where she was and I drove the twenty minute journey to the large country house, wondering what 'get me out' meant. When I entered the main bedroom I did not need to wonder any longer.

She was trapped in a position I will take a long time to forget, and cannot fully reveal here. Suffice to say that above her lay the very naked and very dead body of her now ex-lover, and to one side the telephone she had been able to reach with her only free hand.

I released her and together we made our escape, after I had checked the body to make sure he was indeed dead – rather unnecessary, given the circumstances. Natural causes, no doubt, and someone was sure to find him soon. There was nothing to be gained by revealing the full events surrounding his death, and I had no moral or ethical difficulty in just quietly slipping away.

A couple of days later my partner wandered into my consulting room and just stood there, smiling quietly as he does when he's feeling pleased with himself or thinks I have overstepped the mark – or better still, both. I tried to pretend I hadn't noticed he was there, but as usual it didn't bother him at all. He just waited until I put my pen down and sat back in my chair.

'Go on,' I said, 'I can't bear that smug look on your face.'

He smiled even more smugly, the swine, and said, 'I was called out to old Altwhistle the other day by his wife. Came home from a shopping trip and found him dead as a doornail in bed.'

'Really?' I said, feigning boredom.

'Yes, really,' said Philip. God, he could be irritating when he wanted to. 'Nothing unusual about all this of course, apart from the fact that he was naked and his wife said she hadn't seen him without his clothes on for several years. Apparently he would rarely go to bed in the middle of the day, either. Still, the old boy was bound to pop off one day – wrote him up as natural causes, of course, but I just wondered . . . Did you know anything about this, at all?'

I put on my most innocent of faces.

'Me, no, why should I? He was your patient, not mine.'

'Oh, no reason, really. Just wondered.' He turned to open the door and then turned back, took a step towards me and placed something on my desk. 'It's just that you left your stethoscope there, that's all.'

I have an Irish friend whose family are all passionate Rugby Union supporters, never missing an international either live or on TV.

On one memorable occasion the whole family were sitting round one Saturday afternoon watching Ireland versus Wales at Lansdowne Road, Dublin, when my friend's father, a highly excitable man, had a heart attack just before half-time and dropped stone dead on the floor.

'And right in the middle of the game too,' said Lucy ruefully. 'Would you not believe it of him?'

'I would,' I agreed.

'And there he was, all lying there on the floor of the living room and we had to keep stepping over him, too, to fiddle with the reception, so we did.'

When the game was over – 'Well, Dad wouldn't have wanted us to miss the second half now, would he? Specially an Irish win, don't you know' – they summoned the undertaker to perform the necessary duties.

Moving the body proved to be a bit of a problem, as Lucy's parents lived in a second-floor flat and the stairs up to it were too narrow to negotiate a coffin. Eventually the undertaker and his assistant – a young cockney lad – decided to carry the body downstairs themselves, loading it into the coffin at ground-floor level.

All went well from the living room to the top of the stairs, where unfortunately the undertaker lost his footing. He, the body and the undertaker's assistant, who was two steps below tumbled down the entire flight, landing in an entwined heap at the bottom. It took Lucy and her husband Donal a good ten minutes to untangle the assorted limbs.

'Nobody knew quite what to say,' recounted Lucy drily. 'Me poor dead father, missing the end of a grand Irish win and then tumbling down the stairs like that. I ask you, what next indeed? We none of us knew what to say, we did.'

The situation was rescued by the undertaker's assistant, who – freed from his temporary imprisonment – drew himself to his full height and announced in broad cockney, 'Well, you gotta laugh, incha?'

In my early days as a GP – fresh-faced, innocent, idealistic and broke – I received a call from a neighbouring farmer.

'Need ye help,' he said tersely. 'Got a dead body in m' field. Hurry up now – time's money and there's a business to run.'

I drove the few miles to his farm down typically winding Devonian lanes and pulled up in the all but deserted farmyard next to an ambulance, which had somehow managed to get there before me. There was an eerie silence as I stepped out of my car, and the echo as I closed the door reverberated around me.

There was no one in sight.

I stood and listened, wondering in which direction to proceed, when I heard a familiar drone over the horizon. There is to my mind something indescribably sinister about the approach of a helicopter, that most wonderful of flying machines, which probably comes from having seen *Apocalypse Now* once too often after a night out in the local hostelry.

The Cornish Air Ambulance hove into sight, its red bodywork glistening in the bright sunlight, and disappeared from view towards a field a couple of hundred yards to my left. I headed towards it, arriving a few minutes after it had landed next to the milking shed. There before me lay the body of an elderly man in a worn grey suit, surrounded by two air ambulancemen, two ground ambulancemen, the farmer and three of his workers.

They all stood dutifully aside as I approached, no doubt awaiting my expert assessment of the situation. Fresh out of training and with little more than a passing knowledge of procedure and established routine that I have long since both forgotten and ceased to pay any attention to, I decided to take control. One of the ambulancemen was bending over the body.

'Don't touch him,' I snapped peremptorily. 'Unexplained death – it's a coroner's case, don't you understand that? You cannot move the body until you have official permission to do so.'

I was, of course, young, arrogant and cocky, and probably the least proficient in my own field of any of those present.

The ambulancemen passed a look between them, and to their eternal credit stood back without comment on the young upstart before them. I took a deep breath and puffed out my chest importantly, preparing myself to take charge. Just then I noticed an aged farm worker sauntering casually towards us with his dog.

'Stop there,' I ordered. 'We have an unidentified corpse here and already these people have disturbed the scene. Keep your dog back as well. I don't want anything else interfering with this case.'

(Yes, I am cringing as I write this.)

The farmhand regarded me calmly. Reaching into his pocket he slowly and deliberately withdrew his tobacco, rolled a cigarette and lit it with the flick of a wrist.

'Well, young man,' he said in measured country tones, 'that's as maybe. But there's a herd of Friesian cows as needs a-milkin' comin' through 'ere any moment now, an' you, me, the dog an' that there corpse just ain't gonna stop them.'

I looked down at the body, glanced across at my assembled colleagues, and then I considered myself and my pompous, overbearing, self-important attitude. Two of them had to go.

'Right then,' I said with a shame-faced grin. 'Two on the arms, two on the legs, and I suppose I can just about cope with the head myself.'

Of such moments are careers made or broken.

As the loudly mooing herd crested the hill above us, tumbling inexorably into our midst, we lifted the body, and ran for it.

After now some ten years in general practice I know my patients fairly well and have often been intimately acquainted with parts of their bodies neither they nor I would wish to routinely expose in public places. In my early days, however, two and a half thousand patients were relative strangers, whose lives, relationships and homes I had yet to enter.

I have an extremely retentive memory for medical trivia – meet a patient in the street and I could probably tell you when their catheter bag was last changed, what their favourite choice of suppository is, and how they explained that unfortunate accident last

year with a jar of French mustard. But ask me their name and
those of their closest relatives and my mind would become
immediately blank.

So when the phone rang during surgery, interrupting Mrs
Battersby, and my receptionist said in hushed tones, 'It's Mr
Haslett. You know, *that* Mr Haslett,' in fact I didn't, and my mind
instantly slipped into neutral, that happy state of tranquillity
apparently enjoyed by the English cricket team whenever they
venture out on to the field of play these days.

I reserve it for such occasions as when I am serenely watching
the test match on the TV carefully positioned behind my comprehensive library of 'Women's Problems – Your Role In
Understanding Them'. I've never actually read any but they make
a splendid sight screen behind which to view the TV whilst Mrs
Battersby is telling me how she always gets diarrhoea in Margate
and could it be the winkles.

'Oh, that Mr Haslett,' I responded nonchalantly, wondering all
the while whether the English cricket captain would benefit from
some high colonic lavage. 'Do put him through.'

'It's about my wife,' said Mr Haslett, breathing heavily. 'I've
just got her back from hospital, doctor, and I thought you might
like to come round and see her. I'm so grateful to you for sending
her in, I'll never forget what you did for her.'

I had not the least idea who Mr Haslett was, why his wife had
been in hospital, or what it was I was supposed to have done for
her, but I was learning fast.

'You must be so glad to have her home,' I enthused sympathetically. 'A great relief, I'm sure.' I covered the mouthpiece in a
hurry as I punched the air and shouted 'Yes, yes, yes,' as the great
Ian Botham dispatched the ball for the boundary he needed to
reach his century, temporarily oblivious to my surroundings. A
voice came through the haze.

'I'm so glad you agree,' said Mrs Battersby warmly. 'Most
people just don't understand, but a sweat rash can be so awfully

embarrassing at a cocktail party. I can't thank you enough, doctor . . .'

There are times during general practice when I feel I must have inadvertently strayed into a Jack Kerouac novel, and am unable to find the way out. I suddenly realised I was currently engaged in three mutually exclusive exchanges, and the only one I was remotely interested in involved twenty-two men in white shirts. Time to pull myself together and behave like the dedicated and responsible GP I hoped one day I might become.

'I'll be there imminently,' I reassured Mr Haslett. 'It will be nice to see her again.'

I ignored the slightly disconcerting, 'No hurry, doctor. She won't be going anywhere for a couple of days,' and returned to the immediate problem of Mrs Battersby and her social embarrassments.

'Have you considered Aran sweaters?' I suggested helpfully. 'So bulky and all-encompassing . . .'

I propelled the good lady to the door, deaf to her protestations that the wool would give her hives, and returned to the test match. Of such pleasures is general practice made.

Two blissful hours later – admittedly only at the end of play for the day – the spectre of Mr Haslett and his recently discharged wife returned to my mind. 'Discharge', I always feel, is one of those unfortunate words that just begs to be misinterpreted. When somebody tells me that their nearest and dearest has just been 'discharged' from hospital it conjures up a picture of a human cannonball being forcibly expelled from the depths of the hospital basement and flying through the air before coming to land somewhere in the Devonian hinterlands.

I resolved to visit Mrs Haslett. Whoever she was, she would no doubt be pleased to see me, whilst her husband – who obviously already held me in the highest esteem for a service I could not recall rendering – would likely spread the gospel of my devotion to the cause and unfailing concern for those who placed their delicate health in my sure-footed hands.

Just what a new young doctor needs as he tries to build up his reputation. It was a no lose situation.

In the event, Mrs Haslett was entirely uninterested in my presence. Her husband answered the door in dressing gown and slippers, looking rather grey and careworn. Poor chap's worn out with all the worry, I thought, overflowing with unaccustomed empathy.

'And how is Mrs Haslett?' I asked breezily. 'Glad to be back, I trust?'

He stared at me somewhat blankly.

'I suppose she would be glad to be home, if you put it that way, doctor,' he said in a faltering voice. 'She's in the sitting room. Should I show you through?'

Mrs Haslett was indeed in the sitting room, just as he had said. She was also very dead.

In an old-fashioned country tradition I had not previously encountered, he had brought her home to lie in state and invited his new, caring young doctor to come and pay his respects.

I duly paid them, and fled.

Every now and then, however, we wander into a world of the bizarre, the eerie or the frankly surreal.

I was called out one day by the local police to certify a death. This sometimes happened in my then capacity as the local police surgeon, usually to establish whether there were suspicious circumstances or not. On other occasions it would be simply because one of my patients had died and they just needed some formal identification together with confirmation that life was indeed extinct.

It was a welcome diversion on this occasion as I was busily explaining to the inexhaustible lady before me for the third time that week that no, I didn't actually want her to die, but it would save the NHS in general and me in particular a considerable amount of time, energy and money if she did. We would all miss her terribly, of course, when her demise actually occurred, but in the meantime perhaps she could manage to be a little less of a burden to our ever-diminishing budget.

The police, of course – just like ourselves – are not always over-endowed with the jelly-like substance between the ears. I was once called to confirm a death in a man who had expired at least two days previously, but they thought he was perhaps alive because the body was still warm. Of course it was – he was lying in bed with the electric blanket full on.

Another day or two and he would have been dry roasted.

You do get used to death as a GP, even occasionally rather blasé. It's all part of a day's work, sadly enough, but I was a little upset on this particular occasion because the man concerned, a widower in his early sixties, had only recently lost his wife. She had been bedridden for many years, throughout which time he had devotedly and assiduously nursed her, no doubt sometimes guiltily wondering how he was best going to enjoy his freedom when it ultimately came.

It seemed unfair that he should die so soon, and I just hoped he had packed in a whole load of unashamed hedonistic activity in the preceding few months.

I drew up to the house, in a quiet cul-de-sac in modest suburbia, noticing the police car outside in the drive.

Must be inside, I thought.

I had not actually spoken to the police myself – we employ receptionists to deal with the public whenever possible, you understand – and therefore sauntered casually into the house with not the least idea of what I was about to find.

The first thing I found was the smell, about five yards short of the front door. The smell of death, but also the smell of something else. Something I could not immediately define until I stepped into the hall and remembered that my ex-patient had a dog, and that if the patient was dead, his dog would not be able to open the door to the garden to attend to his natural ablutions. It transpired,

Death in Strange Places

in fact, that he had not been able to do that for the past five days, but I was blissfully ignorant of this minor detail until a little later.

'Hello,' I called, rather feebly to be honest, and, 'Hello,' again. Now I do know that dead patients are rather limited in their conversation, but most policemen can cope with a simple greeting on their good days.

Silence. I manoeuvred my way carefully down the hall – the dog, remember – and entered the back bedroom of the bungalow more by instinct than because I had any knowledge of where my late patient might be. The room, like the rest of the house, was in darkness.

Have you ever noticed how, in all the best thrillers, the heroine wanders around the house in the presence of the suspected intruder, heated curlers in hand, and never ever turns the light on?

'Turn the light on, you stupid woman,' I always want to bellow, 'and then you'll see him standing by the kitchen knives wondering which one will do the job most effectively.'

But they never do, and for some reason I did not either.

So there I was, in the bedroom of a deserted house, in the gloom and the smell and the silent eeriness of it all, knowing that there were two of us present and I was the only one still breathing. Yet still I had not turned a light on. I took a deep breath, regretted it, and illuminated the scene.

Now I am not a squeamish man – I'm a doctor, and we are trained, eager, willing and thoroughly prepared for every eventuality (complete falsehood, of course, but it sounds good) – but even I recoiled at the sight which met my eyes.

My patient was lying in bed, completely unrecognisable. I think it was the shock of not expecting to see what I did that made it so much worse. I assumed he had just died and would look like the man I remembered, which in fact is probably exactly what he did look like – a small matter of five days previously.

His entire body had turned black and swollen monstrously to more than three times its normal size. His abdomen was grossly

202

distended, and had macabrely strained his pyjama top to such an extent that some of the buttons had burst off, whilst those still remaining looked unequal to the job in hand. His head was bloated beyond recognition and a trail of dried blood had solidified from the corner of his mouth to the floor.

My senses reeling, I just stood there, incapable of movement, feeling for a moment I must have strayed into a Hammer horror movie by mistake. I was just thinking that any moment now Peter Cushing would appear round the corner carrying a wooden stake when I heard footsteps approach. I clutched the nearest thing to hand and then realising exactly what it was clutched something else instead whilst I waited, rooted to the spot.

To my relief, a policeman stuck his head round the door, and came tentatively in. 'Just been out for some air,' he said weakly.

I still cannot see a policeman without wondering if I have paid my car tax within the past six months, or if they have finally caught up with me for cherry knocking at Mrs Ecclestone's house on my way home from junior school, but for once I was very glad to see one of the men in blue, particularly as he looked even more awful than I was currently feeling.

We stood in contemplation of the body together, transfixed, sharing the same feeling.

Nausea.

'Pretty awful,' he said eventually.

I nodded my agreement, and we looked some more, unable somehow to leave the horror of the scene.

And then it happened. There was a gurgling sound from the body. We glanced across at each other, pale and aghast, before slowly, inexorably, our gaze was drawn back towards the corpse. More gurgling, then without warning the dried blood in his mouth liquefied and burst forth in a torrent down his chin, like an extinct volcano reactivating. It was awful enough, but there was more to come.

The accumulated gases in his stomach rumbled and churned,

the strain on the final two buttons of his pyjama jacket reached breaking point. Finally the pressure was too great and they flew off like a couple of rifle shots in the stillness, one speeding towards the light and smashing the bulb, leaving us in complete, startling darkness.

We were trained, experienced professionals, so we did what all trained, experienced professionals would do in such adverse circumstances.

We turned tail and ran.

So death can be peaceful, moving, undignified, funny and sometimes surreal or bizarre. In my early days, whilst still in the air force and not fully trained as a GP, I was doing a locum for my practice-to-be. This was of course mostly for the money, but partly as a trial run to see whether I would ultimately be suitable to join. The incumbent GP was away on holiday, and I was entirely on my own for a few days.

The telephone rang at about six a.m. on a beautiful summer's morning and I answered it with a degree of trepidation. It was the first time I had been left completely alone to deal with whatever came my way, there being nobody else to turn to for advice.

I was less than fully confident of my ability to cope.

'Dr Sparrow,' came a brisk female voice of the horses, dogs and wellington boots brigade.

'Yes?' I said guardedly.

'Need you. Problems here. Straight down the road, first left, you'll see me.'

'What's the problem?' I asked cautiously. I had been taught to always prepare for what you might find. There was a grunt of irritation at the other end of the phone.

'Problem – problem is you're not moving quick enough. Come, man. Patient trying to kill herself. Throwing herself in front of cars, that sort of thing. Hurry please – can't stop her for ever.'

The phone went dead. Oh dear! I thought. I wasn't ready for this at all.

I found my patient, Ellen – who looked eerily like Heidi as a great-grandmother – sitting down on the kerbside of the A30, which was then the major road from Devon into Cornwall but is now just a sleepy village street.

Having arrived not so much at the scene of the crime as the scene of the scene, so to speak, I returned to my basic training (even I had some, little enough though it was) and took stock of the situation.

It didn't help at all. I still didn't know what to do.

Gradually, however, the story unfolded. Heidi – not her real name, but I cannot think of her as any other – was a recluse who had scarcely been seen in the village for several years. Her husband was even more of a recluse – he hadn't been seen at all.

There were doubts, apparently, as to whether he actually existed and I suppose at this precise moment those doubts could be said to be well founded. Heidi hadn't seen him for two days, and thought he must be dead. She therefore decided to kill herself as she couldn't manage without him and showing great presence of mind headed for the main road, seeking out the largest heavy goods vehicle she could find.

Along had come Mrs Horse, Dogs and Welly, sitting astride the horse, but unfortunately for Heidi the eagerly anticipated HGV was sadly missing, it being only six o'clock in the morning. Trying therefore to seize the only opportunity available to her, with great determination she endeavoured to throw herself under the horse. She missed. You're with me so far? Well, this is where it begins to get interesting.

Her husband, it transpires, was missing, but being a recluse of some stature he was missing back in the house. Heidi was sure he must be in there somewhere, but she could not actually find him. At this point I felt I had wandered inadvertently into a Salvador Dali painting and was unable to find my way out again.

Mrs Horse, Dogs and Welly – HDW for short – took control.
'Perhaps we should go and look for him?' she ventured, which
at the time seemed like a pretty good idea. We had to look for the
house first, Heidi being apparently uncertain exactly where she
had left it, and despite the fact that it was less than four hundred
yards from the surgery it took a lot of finding.

It was surrounded by such dense undergrowth – not to mention a hell of a lot of overgrowth – that even though it was no
more than a few yards from the kerb you could not actually see it
until you almost bumped into it. In fact, although I had driven
past it on many occasions I had been completely unaware of its
existence.

I entered the gloom lying ominously behind the front door and
immediately I too, like Heidi, knew her husband was dead. Death
has an odour all of its own, and I could smell him. The trouble
was I could not see him, or anything else for that matter, so I fum-
bled around inside the hall and switched the light on.

This cunning ploy to ease the forthcoming search was sadly
ineffective, as the electricity had been disconnected sometime in
the previous decade, but gradually my eyes became accustomed to
the dark and I began my macabre search. The house was packed
to the brim with years of yellowing newspapers, hundreds of cardboard boxes and enough saucepans – not all of them empty – to
stock a chain of hardware stores for the best part of a generation.

Slowly I worked my way from one end of the house to the
other, scattering cardboard boxes in my wake. There was no husband to be found anywhere, though I sensed his presence. I beat
a tactical withdrawal, emerging into the brilliant sunshine and
shading my eyes.

'I, er, can't find him,' I proffered weakly.

Heidi muttered something indistinct to Mrs HDW, who
looked at me as if she had just discovered her sense of humour for
the first time in many years.

'She says, "Have you tried upstairs?"' she translated calmly, and indeed I had not. This was not due to any lack of fortitude or diligence on my behalf – I had not looked upstairs because I had not actually found a staircase.

I re-entered the house with my heart no longer sinking – it had sunk as low as it could possibly reach, and there was nowhere else for it to sink to. I found the stairs, eventually, concealed – yes, you've guessed it – beneath a truly monstrous pile of cardboard boxes. Climbing the stairs was simple – I picked up the cardboard boxes in front of me, threw them over my shoulder and ascended each step one at a time.

Ten minutes later, I stood at the top of the stairs. I still could not see them, buried as they were beneath the cardboard wake I had created, but Edmund Hillary himself could have felt no more triumphant as he crested the 29,000th foot of Mount Everest.

I found Heidi's husband, who was very dead indeed, in one of the bedrooms. The smell was overpowering, and unable to face the return route I left courtesy of an upstairs window and a convenient drainpipe. The rest of the morning passed in a blur.

Heidi was eventually taken away to the local psychiatric hospital, under a section, which seems a sensible option but was in fact illegal, because to prevent her running away again, Mrs HDW made her a cup of tea and I made her a Mickey Finn. When the psychiatric social worker arrived to assess her condition Heidi was fast asleep and then some.

You cannot unfortunately section an unconscious patient according to any of the rules we are supposed to abide to.

Still, common sense prevailed and section her we did. I returned to the surgery, feeling I had come of age at last, and sat with a cup of coffee musing on my morning's labours whereupon Mrs HDW appeared and waved a telephone number under my nose.

'Heidi's brother,' she announced in a matter of fact manner. 'Thought you might like to give him a ring.'

How she acquired the number I have not the least idea, but

with a heavy heart I rang and explained all to Heidi's only living relative.

There was a silence at the end of the phone. Poor chap, I thought, he's overcome with the emotion of it all. And then he spoke.

'Sorry, mate,' he said, 'not much I can do about it, I'm afraid. Just off on me holidays – packing the car when you rang. Deal with it all, will you, and tell Heidi I'll give her a ring when I get back.'

The phone went dead, and I was left looking at the receiver with a mix of unusual emotions.

A year after this bizarre event the land was cleared. For the first time you could properly see the house, now very attractively refurbished. To everyone's surprise an equally attractive barn, now expensively converted, was also unearthed.

Two other new houses have since been built on the land they owned, which was more extensive than anyone expected. Heidi's brother, he who was too intent upon his holiday to help in any way, must have profited to the tune of nearly half a million pounds.

I hope he enjoys every penny of it.

11

Not an Everyday Occurrence

Some of your patients live on in the mind long after they have left the practice, be it vertically or horizontally.

Take Jacob Markstow, for example.

Jacob loved taking tablets. Or to be more precise, he loved taking medication and then complaining about the side effects from it, the more debilitating the better.

He collected unusual responses, nurtured them like children, encouraged them, welcomed them into his life to recount whenever the opportunity arose with a touching combination of sheer delight and childish hurt that he should be the innocent victim of such repetitive iatrogenic misfortune.

Most evenings would find him in the Fox and Grapes, tweed jacket straining vainly to meet round whatever particularly virulent choice of waistcoat he had decided to bless his audience with that day. Elbow resting solidly on the bar, ruddy cheeks quivering with emotion, he would recall to all within earshot the latest assault on his poor, ailing body by that torturer incarnate, his GP.

That is . . . me.

'Bloody man, said it would make me arthritis better, and it might a bit at that, but look at me, just look at me, wasting away I am,' he would say, tapping his great rotund abdomen in apparent despair, 'wasting away. That bloody doctor, causes me more problems with 'is there bloody tablets than I ever 'ad before I went to see 'im in the first place. I ask yer, I bloody ask yer . . .'

'So why do you take them?' somebody asked him politely.

'Well, I needs them, don't I?' replied Jacob, bridling with

indignation and stretching up to his full five foot six in height. 'Enough bloody tablets in the world. Even *he's* got to get it right, sooner or later.'

He always had a captive audience for his tales of woe, partly – to be fair – because he could be an engaging companion, had no real malice within him and was blessed with a rich fund of stories about country life. He was also extremely well off and could be relied upon to more than stand his round for anybody who was listening, which in practice was usually everyone in the bar at the time.

I swear I once heard him say, 'Went right through me, they did, went right through me,' after I had prescribed him some glycerine suppositories. This, I admit, was in a fit of purely professional revenge at the end of a typically long-winded consultation. Jacob always described his symptoms in as vague and imprecise a manner as possible, and on this occasion had hinted that he might possibly perhaps have been a little shy of the bathroom lately.

The thought of Jacob inserting the suppositories in the appropriate orifice one night only to vomit them up the next morning, and the actual mode of transit, would divert me in many an idle moment. It became particularly useful during tedious consultations when I had long since switched off and stopped listening to what the patient had to say.

Our consultations were generally uneasy compromises – in other words he got precisely what he wanted whilst I uneasily compromised.

'Oh, but surely,' he would say beseechingly, 'surely you're not going to refuse to treat me? You must have something new and expensive you can give me.'

Price mattered to Jacob. A state of the art, brand new blood pressure pill, fresh off the presses and costing as much as his shiny new tractors, that could give him a bout of the collywobbles, would keep him in mournful complaints for weeks at a time.

'It's not entirely your fault it so often goes wrong, and I am in *so* much pain.'

'OK, Jacob,' I would inevitably concede. 'How could I deny you the opportunity to react badly to something new?'

But sarcasm was wasted, on him.

He came to see me one morning smiling benignly.

'Easy one for you today, doc. Just need my ears syringing.'

What he kindly did not say, although we both knew he could, was that even I might be hard pressed to mess it up this time.

I inspected his ears, and somewhat to my surprise they really did need a major washout. I suggested we soften the wax first, both to make the actual event a little easier and to delay the inevitable aftermath of complaint, whatever that might ultimately be.

And there would be something, of that I was certain.

He wanted me to syringe them there and then. I stalled for a moment, realised the hopelessness of my position, and set to work resignedly. It didn't work, and it made him dizzy. Then it made him nauseous, and finally he developed a transient but totally disabling sensation that his entire body was on fire.

I gave him an ear wax softener, and promised him it would work without fail.

He came back a week later and I tried again. To our collective dismay it didn't work, and made his ears itch. I gave him some olive oil, but that didn't work either, giving him pins and needles in his 'middle, somewhere in me middle.'

'Middle of what?' I inquired forlornly.

'Middle of *me*,' he countered belligerently.

I gave up and decided to go for broke. Making up some sodium bicarbonate drops I labelled it 'The Mixture' and gave it to him with a ceremonial flourish. He studied it intently.

'Any side effects?'

'None whatsoever,' I replied firmly.

'You're sure?' he persisted.

There are times in general practice, just as indeed there are times in life, when you look back and say to yourself, 'Why did I do that?'

This was one of them. 'Well,' I began, unable to resist, 'it may make your water turn green.'

Oh, the things we do say when we are under pressure. His eyes lit up with delight, his cheeks shining with pleasure. I could see he was already working on his next story for the willing audience in the Fox and Grapes.

He came back a week later.

'It won't work, doc,' he said dolefully. 'My water is as clear as crystal.'

'It will,' I reassured him. 'Perhaps this is just the one side effect you are destined not to have. Unlike Mrs . . .' I added wickedly.

I allowed my voice to tail off, catching the fleeting sense of disappointment on his face as he no doubt resolved to do better.

He had the most stubborn wax in Christendom. In desperation I thought quickly. 'Jacob,' I said, 'did I tell you it only goes green if you leave it to stand overnight?'

'Never mentioned it,' he replied, his eyes beginning to light up again.

Three days later he came back a sad and dejected man. I syringed his ears easily until they were beautifully clean, explaining to him what a good job I had done.

'M'be, doctor,' he replied, crestfallen. 'But it obviously wasn't that mixture of yours,' he added, brightening a little. 'My water is still as clear as clear can be.'

'It can take several days,' I consoled him. 'Just give it one more try for me, tonight.'

He nodded his head meekly, and promised he would.

My telephone rang at six o'clock the next morning, not long after I had come in from an early call.

'It's wonderful,' burbled Jacob. 'Just wait till I tell them this down at the pub. It's as green as green can be.'

212

So if you should ever meet him, down at the Fox and Grapes with his elbow on the bar and jacket buttons straining fit to bust, you'll notice him fingering his left pocket ostentatiously. At the merest suggestion of interest on your behalf he will bring out his bottle full of green urine and place it reverentially on the bar before you.

'I'll tell you a story . . .' he'll say.

I no longer mind about Jacob. I feel at peace with the world.

That early morning visit I had been on?

In Devon, to the amazement of our friends from the city, we often leave our back doors unlocked when we go out, let alone in. Indeed, I once went on holiday for two weeks and left the back door not only unlocked but wide open, and on returning home was disappointed to find that nobody had been in to tidy up a bit in my absence. But back to Jacob.

At 5.30 a.m. I had crept into his house through the unlocked back door, into the kitchen and quietly out again, clutching my bottle of green vegetable dye close to my heart.

It is a churlish thought, and one that I am inveterately rather ashamed of, but I have no doubt that most, if not all, of my colleagues have shared it at one moment or another in their careers – patients will die at the most inconvenient of times.

You can prowl the hospital corridors, waiting for that final moment, the seemingly penultimate breath, that last deep gasp before they gently slide unseen into another world . . . then suddenly they open their eyes and ask for a cup of tea. Irritated at their perversity you decide it will be another few hours or so before they die, and you return to the surgery.

When you get there the receptionist is holding the phone, waiting for you.

'It's the hospital,' she says, biting her lip as she waits for you to react. 'Mrs Abernathy died two minutes after you left them.'

It sounds callous, inhuman and uncaring, especially when that flare of irritation hits you. But it is not that – death is part of our way of life, and we have to learn to cope with the loss of a patient without it affecting our ability to deal with the next. The adjustment, the rationalisation and the emotional reassessment come later, in a quiet moment.

So when my receptionist buzzed me at five to nine on a Monday morning to tell me that old Mrs Edwards' next-door neighbour had found her dead at the bottom of the stairs, I hope you will begin to understand why my first emotion was one of extreme irritation. Why should she die now, when I had a full waiting room and three visits already to undertake? Why couldn't the neighbour have waited until lunchtime to go and visit her?

Why had she registered with me anyway when she lived so far away?

All these appallingly irreverent thoughts vanished in but a second as I spoke to an obviously distressed middle-aged lady who had just seen her first dead body and was struggling unevenly to come to terms with the situation. I put the phone down, apologised to the waiting room, explaining I had an urgent call to attend, and drove off into the countryside, drawing up at the small rundown end terrace cottage with a heavy heart. She had been a dear old lady, Mrs Edwards, grateful for the smallest assistance and always eager to press a cup of tea upon you, or a newly baked scone.

She had been due to go into hospital today for a hip replacement, and hopefully a new lease of life free from the pain that had nagged her for the past ten years. It was too late for that, now.

I went next door, to find three middle-aged ladies sitting down, mugs of tea in hand, gently commiserating with each other over the tragedy that had entered their day.

'Hello,' I said, feeling a little inadequate as I intruded into their private grief. 'I'm . . .'

The nearest of the three turned to look at me, an expression of mixed relief and despair etched on her plump face.

'. . . Dr Sparrow,' she finished for me. 'Yes, we know who you are, dear.'

'It was just so sudden,' burst in the lady to her right, a small, thin weathered woman so typical of the school of hard knocks in this rural backwater. 'Poor old Kath, she was so looking forward to . . .'

She dissolved in quiet tears, and again that feeling of helpless inadequacy washed over me. Whatever I did, whatever I said, it would not ease the pain of the loss of one of their own.

I excused myself and squelched through the mud to the house next door. The ambulance had arrived in the interim, and reversed into the narrow drive, the engine idling somewhat obtrusively in the still country air. I opened the back door and stepped into a world I felt more comfortable with.

'Hello, doc,' said the younger of the two ambulancemen, a man I had met many times in the past few years. 'Getting a cup of tea while we do all the work for you?'

In our part of the world we are blessed with some of the finest ambulancemen/paramedics you could wish to see anywhere. Thin on the ground they may be, but proficient, unfailingly cheerful despite some of the appalling circumstances in which we often meet, and professional beyond belief.

I have no idea as to the respective feelings of our patients when they see both ambulance and doctor arrive. Tradition, I suspect, dictates that our charges breathe a sigh of relief when the doctor's car pulls up outside their front door which is almost – but not quite – as deep as the breath we will take when we realise the ambulance has got there before us. We need them for their expertise far more often than they need us for ours.

'Nice of you to turn up,' I responded, 'and on the same day you were called, as well. Things are looking up.'

'We wouldn't have bothered, had it been your partner,' came

the deadpan response, 'but he doesn't need us to hold his hand like you do. He actually appears to know what he is doing.'

'I love you too,' I replied, 'it's just I love some of the others of you more than yourselves.'

They grinned, relaxed and confident in their undoubted expertise, and we turned our attention to the task in hand.

Mrs Edwards was lying crossways at the bottom of the stairs, and it was hard to be sure precisely what had happened. Had she tumbled from the top, and met an accidental death, or merely reached the end of the flight and succumbed to natural causes? I still have no idea, and we decided between us that the coroner should be equally unaware.

'Post-mortem won't bring her back,' muttered Jeffrey, the elder of the two.

I nodded my agreement and walked across to where the body lay. The pathos of the situation struck me at last, and my knees – which never give way these days, but remind me occasionally they are still there – buckled slightly.

I looked at the small, frail body, lying across the door mat, and then something caught my eye. To the left of her head, incongruously placed as if just waiting for a tube of Dentucreme to come bursting through the letter box, lay her false teeth, bare and unrepentant in their nakedness.

We would never know – had she been carrying them down in her hands, ready for cleaning prior to breakfast, or had the force of her fall ejected them on to the carpet for us to see, and wonder?

I cannot see a set of false teeth, these days, no matter what the environment, without my mind taking me back to Mrs Edwards, her cups of tea and newly baked scones, and her body lying at the bottom of the stairs, having risen in search of a new dawn.

I often wonder if she found a better one than she had anticipated, and I hope with all my heart that she did.

A life in the world of medicine will inevitably bring you face to face with some of the great ethical problems of our time. Should euthanasia be legalised? How far down the road should we proceed with genetic engineering? Is constipation funny?

And most thought-provoking of all – what do you do when you stumble across a complete cock-up that nobody else has noticed, and probably never will?

It was a routine Monday morning surgery. The waiting room was full, it was drizzling outside, someone had parked in my personal space – again – and old Mrs Petheridge was in her usual corner, wheezing asthmatically. Mondays, Wednesdays and Thursdays she came to the surgery, so regularly that I sometimes wondered if I had actually employed her somewhere along the line and just forgotten about it.

I was never quite sure how she occupied the rest of her week, between appointments – 'Sorry, dear, can't come to the wedding. The doctors will be expecting me . . .' – but she was a dear old thing, and I never minded seeing her. I swear she's going to die there, one day, in her own reserved seat in the corner, and she's probably requested that her ashes be scattered over the waiting-room carpet.

My partner, who had been on call for the weekend, glanced up briefly. 'Saw one of yours on Saturday,' he said absently. 'Old Emily Balsdon. Died in the Methodist church attending her husband's funeral. Right in the middle of Psalm 163.' He grinned wickedly. 'Seemed such a shame to move her. They could have just popped her in another coffin and started the service again, two for the price of one.'

'Go wash your mouth out, young man,' I replied in mock horror. 'Still, poor old Emily. She'd have been lost without her Eddie.'

Emily and Eddie were a delightful elderly couple who lived in a little cottage not far from the surgery. Although frail and arthritic, they both had a sparkling sense of humour and retained a keen interest in life. They had been next-door neighbours and childhood sweethearts, married for nigh on seventy years, and had

217

always hoped to die together, knowing that each would have been devastated to be left alone without the other.

'By the way, she's for cremation too,' added my partner, 'so you'll have to go and view the body. I couldn't do the death certificate, but I knew you would be able to.'

There are strict rules about signing a death certificate. You must of course be confident of the cause of death, it must be anticipated and not sudden and unexpected, and you must have seen the patient yourself within the previous fortnight. Emily had chronic heart failure, and it was no surprise to me that she had succumbed at such a poignant moment.

Her body had been transferred to one of the undertakers in the local town. For a body to be cremated, the certifying doctor has to physically see the deceased himself – for a burial, confirmation of death by any old doctor will do.

I rang the funeral director, Peter Sandercock, whom I knew well. 'Hi, Peter, it's Mike Sparrow. Look, I'm a bit busy today, do you mind if I leave it till tomorrow to come and see Emily's body?'

'That'll be fine, Mike,' he said. 'Funeral's not until Thursday, and the family have all paid their respects. I'll probably not see you, we've got a busy few days – three funerals today, two tomorrow.'

'Quite a turnover,' I agreed. 'Business is obviously booming.'

'Well, we enjoy it while it lasts,' he replied philosophically. 'Can't go round hoping for too many deaths, can we? Let yourself in, when you get here. You've still got your own key, haven't you?'

Because I generally visited his emporium at the end of the working day, he had given me a key in case the building was unmanned – save for the corpses, of course, who in general were unable to open the doors for you.

Most undertakers have a chilled room on the premises where the bodies – and in the summer, cold drinks – are kept awaiting further disposal. Mr Sandercock had an 'Arthur Daley' lock-up situated down a quiet back street some distance from his main office.

I always found it an eerie experience opening up the deserted building and walking deferentially through the still and the quiet to where three large heavy doors stood before you. Behind each was a 'cooler', with five rows of sliding metal frames on which the bodies lay. Each could be drawn out on smoothly running rollers, for admission, discharge or, just like me, viewing purposes.

I arrived late the next evening and wondered through the dark ghostly environs, and opened the first door in the quest for poor old Emily. Five pairs of cold feet were arrayed vertically before me, each with a handwritten label looped around the big toe. Second from the top I could read 'Emily Balsdon, RIP . . .' and the date.

I pulled out the tray, rolled down the sheet, and stopped, frozen to the spot. Whoever was lying in that particular section was an imposter. Emily Balsdon it was not.

I checked the label on her big toe, and 'Emily Balsdon' it said again. I looked back at the body, just in case a major transformation had suddenly taken place, but it was no more Emily now than it had been a minute earlier. I pushed the shelf back in on its rollers and stood thinking for a moment, and then systematically checked the other four bodies in the column.

None of them were Emily either, or even a passable imitation, so I frantically opened the other two sections, neither of which was completely full, and checked the remaining seven bodies one by one. I took a deep breath, exhaling slowly, and sat down with all twelve bodies exposed before me, thinking very carefully what I should do next.

All that kept coming into my mind were the words of Peter Sandercock. 'We've got a busy few days – three funerals today, two tomorrow.'

'Emily,' I murmured to myself. 'Oh Emily, where art thou?'

Half an hour later I was sitting before an ashen-faced Peter in

219

the quiet seclusion of his study. Emily Balsdon, whose ashes were due to be buried next to her husband in two days' time, had today been cremated before a group of grieving friends and relatives – none of them actually her own – and then solemnly interred next to a complete stranger.

To his eternal credit, Peter never once thought of himself and the effect on his business reputation of this ghastly state of affairs. His sympathies were only with the families, and the suffering that was bound to follow.

'I can't see any other option,' he said finally. 'We don't have any choice, we have to tell them.'

I was just about to agree with him when a vision of Emily came into my mind. I was sitting one bitterly cold winter's morning in their kitchen, warming my hands round a cup of tea and enjoying the heat from the old Rayburn as it spread into my back.

They had just celebrated their sixty-eighth wedding anniversary, and were keenly anticipating their seventieth, as much in love with each other as ever before.

'And do you know,' said Emily warmly, resting her wrinkled hand gently on her husband's shoulder as he dozed quietly beside her, 'in all that time I have never once looked at another man, let alone lain with one.'

And then much to my surprise, she leaned forward and whispered conspiratorially, 'But I've often wondered what it would be like,' and she gave me a broad wink before sitting back, a gentle smile playing on her lips.

We buried an empty coffin, suitably weighted, in Emily's grave. The family never knew. On a quiet evening, with the much appreciated assistance of an understanding colleague, we cremated the other body and collected the ashes.

And then, in the early hours of the following morning – like a latter-day Burke and Hare – we disinterred Emily's ashes from their temporary resting place, and buried the others in their stead.

Two hours later, Emily was duly returned to her rightful position at her husband's side.

Should we ever have done it? Maybe not, but to this day nobody knows, and nobody grieves, and nobody has suffered as a result of an awful mistake.

And Emily? Well, she had had her secret wish without ever betraying her husband.

She had finally lain with another man.

Agatha, bless her, was not in control of her teeth. Her husband, Frederick, was no longer in control of anything, having died (probably much to his secret relief) a couple of years earlier.

They had lived – and Agatha still did – in a remote tied cottage some distance from the surgery and had an interesting interpersonal relationship. There was none. The house was nominally split in two, and each inhabited their own half exclusively. As Frederick had the half with the bathroom, and Agatha that with the kitchen, it did make you wonder.

I, for one, never had the nerve to ask.

They never spoke directly to each other, as far as I am aware, but ranted vituperatively about their other half to any visitor whom they could persuade to listen. They each had their own separate entrances, and woe betide you if you inadvertently knocked on the wrong door.

The dividing line between their two respective halves was a piece of string nailed lengthwise along the floor of the living room. You would often find them both in there, rigidly adhering to their own side, with two television sets (and invariably two different programmes) blaring forth. The district nurse, visiting one day to give them both their flu jabs, made the mistake of simply stepping across the string from one to the other.

Wrong move. You had to walk out of the front door of the one, around the overgrown path bordering the outside of the house, and in though the front door of the other (there was no 'back' door, each insisting their own entrance was the original) to return to the room you had just left, but now on the correct side of the string.

I was unsure as to whether Agatha's teeth had never fitted, were made for another party, or were just one final memento of her late husband that she could not bear to be parted from. In her way I am sure that she misses him still – the string remains, and she never once transgresses on to his side, but I catch her looking wistfully across to his corner, once in a while.

For all that, her teeth rumbled around in her mouth with a life of their own, making her conversation all but impossible to comprehend. It was most disconcerting – I would spend entire consultations waiting for either or both dentures to reject their host and come flying out on to my desk. It was one of life's unexplained mysteries that they never did.

Agatha was found unconscious at home one day, and my partner thought she had had a stroke. He admitted her to hospital, putting up a subcutaneous (under the skin) drip, more as a 'just in case' measure than with any realistic anticipation of contributing to her survival.

The local geriatrician saw her the next day, and thought she had had a stroke too. I saw her the day after that, and agreed with them both. For four days Agatha lay completely comatose, and for four days we waited for her to die.

We took the drip down, after a collective agreement with her family, and on the fifth day the nurses began tentatively to clear her room. Even the undertaker was aware of her imminent demise. And then as one of the nurses went out to empty her catheter bag, Agatha, who had not moved a muscle on her own for the past five days, suddenly sat bolt upright in bed and bellowed, 'Where's me buggering teeth?'

Despite two sheepish GPs and an even more sheepish consultant, Agatha was none the worse for her experience and survives still. We have no idea what was really wrong with her, or what heralded her startling recovery. She even has a new set of teeth that for the moment, at least, appear to fit.

But I cannot erase the memory of the discarded set, and whenever I see her I remain transfixed upon her mouth, waiting for action.

Patients can be every bit as callous as ourselves, sometimes.

I was round at the farmhouse of a well-known and very large farming family in the area, where the head of the household – an indomitable matriarchal figure in her mid-eighties – was busy breathing her last in an upstairs bedroom, surrounded by innumerable members of her family.

It was a scene reminiscent of those gloriously silly TV programmes I can recall from my youth – how many policemen can you cram in a phone box, how many members of the Mothers' Union can you crush into a Mini – and in this case, how many concerned relatives can actually be holding her hand when she finally dies?

I found the whole thing rather nauseating, I have to say, and was in many ways glad when poor old Gladys finally breathed her last. I made my escape after suitable mumblings and commiserations and wandered down the stairs, leaving everybody trying to outsob each other in the grief department. I opened the door just as the bell rang, and on the doorstep I almost ran into a small wizened man in filthy overalls whom I knew to be from the neighbouring farm.

To my surprise, as he was renowned for his complete absence of generosity, he held in his gnarled and disgusting hands a bottle of very expensive whisky.

'It's for Glad,' he wheezed with a sickly grin. 'Wife said she could be a-doin' of it, time like this.'

My heart softened. There was a spark of humanity in this unedifying specimen of *Homo sapiens* after all. I did not actually warm to him – sort of lukewarmed – and said, 'Look, Albert, I'm sorry to have to tell you this but Gladys has just died. Only a minute or two ago.'

He took a step back and I realised it must have been a bit of a shock to him. But I realised wrong.

A sly grin spread across his face.

'So,' he said thoughtfully, holding the bottle of whisky tight, 'she'll no longer be a-needin' o' this, then, will she?'

It is not every day one of your patients is abducted by aliens.

Of all the patients who have left a lasting impression on me, Alan Jenkinson stands out on his own, a man whose departure from this world I can never forget.

Alan was that rare entity, a Scotsman who had made his life in the West Country, and actually enjoyed it. He was the most honest man I knew – just as well, in view of the fact he was also my bank manager – kind, generous to a fault, and even had a sense of humour.

He was rarely ill, and scarcely ever attended the surgery.

'Too mean to pay a prescription charge,' he would reply with a twinkle in his eye whenever I nagged him about having his blood pressure checked. 'All that banking is not good for a man.'

We had become friends after I removed what appeared to be an innocuous mole from his back some five years earlier, only for it to turn out to be the dreaded malignant melanoma. Happily, he had remained supremely fit and well ever since, showing no sign of succumbing to the unfortunate sequelae of the dreaded disease.

He owned a small farm in the area which I passed each evening on my way home from work, stopping off for a drink on a regular basis. Of course, one drink invariably turned into two, possibly even three, and we would often chat until the early hours. Alan was married but had no children, and although he never referred to it directly I always felt he regretted it, deep down.

For all that, he never once mentioned what I already knew, that his wife was unable to conceive due to a longstanding gynaecological problem. They made an odd couple – his wife, attractive though she was, was dour to the point of apparent rudeness, and they lived fairly independent lives. Despite this, they seemed outwardly happy together, and it was not for me to wonder . . .

I called in one day, on a beautiful late spring evening, expecting to find Alan as usual pottering good-humouredly in his cattle shed, or riding his tractor up and down some already well-ploughed field just for the sheer pleasure of it.

'Smell the land,' he used to say. 'Feel the soil. Go on, Mike, shed the disinfected sterility of that surgery of yours, and remind yourself what real life is all about. Get your hands dirty for once.'

I smelled the land. 'Pig with a hint of silage,' I opined. I felt the soil. 'Just like the stuff in my garden,' I remarked, 'only you've got more of it, and the soap and water's further away.'

'You're just a Philistine,' he grinned.

'But a clean one,' I agreed, 'and I'm proud to say I don't own a single set of overalls, and the only time my wellies have ever had cow manure on them is when I loaned them to you for a week.'

He did have a point, however, and gradually I became seduced by the lure of the land. There was something eerily hypnotic in walking through a field of full-grown corn in the fading light, the evening wind whipping the golden ears against you. Just the sky, the earth, the elements . . . and the smell of silage.

Seduction only goes so far.

This particular evening Alan was not, as usual, clad in wellies, overalls and four different types of mud, but sitting in his study still in his jacket and tie, a pile of magazines scattered on the floor around him. He looked up almost guiltily as I entered.

'No cows to milk?' I asked lightly. 'No lambs to feed, fields to plough, crops to harvest . . . and no glass of Scotch in your hand? Could we be sickening for something?'

He grinned suddenly, and in a split second the Alan I knew was back, although somehow his good humour seemed to sit just a little uneasily on his shoulders.

'Man has to read,' he shrugged, 'and even this man brings his office home once in a while. Come on,' he added as he rose from his chair, guiding me through to the sitting room next door. 'I know the only thing you take home is your proctoscope in case you meet an emergency haemorrhoid along the way, skulking forlornly in some overgrown hedgerow. Got some new home-made wine – not really ready to be drunk, as yet, but we'll be able to appreciate how good it's going to be.'

I looked over my shoulder as we left the study, the heading on an open page of the magazine he had just put down catching my eye.

'UFOs,' I read. 'Why we cannot ignore them.'

The following day I called again. Alan was thankfully back to his normal self, washing down his favourite pig with relish. The pig seemed to be enjoying it almost as much as his owner, grunting and squealing with pleasure.

'But I thought pigs *liked* being dirty,' I said. 'A clean pig is a pig without pleasure.'

'Oh, they do,' he agreed, 'but what they like most is getting seriously filthy just after a good bath. Makes them feel they're in charge, instead of chipolatas in waiting.'

'You don't mean you actually eat them?' I asked, in mock horror.

'Shush,' he admonished, 'he'll hear you.' He nodded to his right. 'Apples doing well in the orchard. They should both be ripe at about the same time. Fancy a trip on my new tractor?'

I did. I just didn't realise he meant a trip to the pub on it . . .

A few weeks later I caught another glimpse of that other Alan. I drove past his house on the way back from branch surgery one lunchtime, and saw his car parked unexpectedly in the drive. He never took a day off work, and it was so unusual I stopped, reversed back, and turned in. The farmhouse was deserted – I rarely saw Alan's wife these days, she either did not like me at all or just had a knack of disappearing, wraith-like, whenever Alan had company.

I strolled around the farmyard and stood looking across the fields, and was just on the point of leaving when I saw a distant figure swaying gently in his field of corn, arms upraised to the heavens. I approached slowly, uneasily, with an uncanny feeling I was about to enter a world I did not understand.

Alan was completely unaware of my approach. He stood in his shirt-sleeves, bare-footed, arms outstretched and reaching to the sky as if beckoning it to come down to him. To his left he had prepared a small clearing, in which the embers of a fire flickered with an odd green light. In front of him lay a small pile of stones, and on top of that a small religious icon that normally resided above the fireplace in his study.

I stood a few yards away, watching and wondering until slowly Alan pivoted and turned to face me. His eyes gradually climbed down from the heavens and came to rest on my face, as if it seemed the most natural thing in the world to find me there.

'They're coming, Mike,' he said, with a childlike simplicity. 'One day, they're coming, and I shall be ready.'

I called in every day, for a while.

Some days I would find the Alan I knew, pig-washing or driving his tractor round a distant field just for the sheer unadulterated hell of it, but at times I would meet the other Alan, lost in a world of his own. Often he would be sitting in his study surrounded by ream after ream of paper covered in scientific drawings beyond my comprehension, with strange hieroglyphics and what seemed to be completely random lines and squiggles punctuated by regularly placed concentric circles and parallelograms.

Let's face it, the guy had gone completely loopy, and I was worried about him. On his rational days I would pursue the point, almost sure he was becoming psychotic, or schizophrenic, or just plain ballistic, but he would chide me gently and resist all input.

'Just my other life,' he would say gently. 'Man cannot live on interest rates, pigs and tractors alone. I'm fine, Mike, you just wouldn't believe me if I told you.'

'Try me,' I suggested. 'I'm very broad-minded. I once had a drink with a Liverpool supporter, for goodness sake. How much more open-minded can a man be?'

'When the time is right,' he would always answer. 'I promise I will tell you when the time is right.'

On the bad days, I just worried. I once bullied a friend of mine, a psychiatrist, to come with me, giving Alan the 'I just happened to be passing, and I've got a friend with me' routine. He was at his most charming and normal – witty, self-effacing and good-humoured.

We stood chatting on the doorstep for a moment as my colleague wandered out to the car, before I bade him farewell.

'Bye, Mike,' he said, patting me gently on the shoulder, 'and say goodbye to your psychiatrist friend for me. Seems like a nice guy.'

'That obvious?' I sighed.

'That obvious,' he nodded.

A few weeks passed. Each time I saw Alan he seemed to snap back into normality and I began to relax, feeling perhaps that the crisis, whatever it might have been, had begun to pass. But I was always on edge, waiting for the next development and hoping it would never come.

It had to happen, sooner or later. A couple of months later I was sitting in my surgery contemplating the forthcoming examination of Mr Hendricks' prostate with less than my customary enthusiasm, when the door burst open and Alan's wife, Maggie, charged into the consulting room like a bull looking for a china shop to run around in. She shuddered to a halt in front of me and stood glowering over my desk.

'He's gone too bloody far, this time,' she hissed venomously, and I wondered how I ever thought that bitterness-etched face could be attractive. 'He's only taken the bloody tractor to work.'

I excused myself quickly – and gratefully – from Mr Hendricks' prostate, and rapidly drove the few miles into the neighbouring town.

Maggie was right. Alan had taken his tractor to work, and then left it there . . .

In his office.

His tractor, polished and gleaming, lay amid the rubble of what used to be the front wall of the bank.

'Interesting piece of parking,' I murmured to a stunned bank teller surveying the debris. 'Has he got a ticket?'

Of Alan there was no sign.

I drove out to the farmhouse. His car was parked in the garage, the front door was open and in some trepidation I slowly entered, fearing and yet not fearing what I might find. I made my way cautiously into the study, looking around me at each step. There on the desk was a glass of whisky, and an envelope bearing my name.

I opened it. *'My dear Mike,'* I read. *'You've probably found the tractor, by now, and I hope enjoyed my parting shot almost as much as did I. I suppose you could say I just wanted to fuse together my two former lives, a coming together of the earth as we know it and that world of grey-suited people I used to inhabit, but actually, it just made a bloody good crash, and I loved it.*

'You'll see a pile of papers on the desk to your left. Read them, and you will understand. The whisky is for you, the one thing I will truly miss about life on earth. I have no real knowledge of what I might find up there, just a sense of excitement like I have never known before.

'Have one last drink with me, Mike. My thanks for your friendship, I will miss that too. I'm only sorry I could not have told you, or you would have had me locked up in a padded room, and thrown away the key.

'*Please don't worry about Maggie, she'll be fine. She won't need to hide her affair any more, and they are welcome to each other, I wish them no harm. Goodbye, Mike, you won't be seeing me again. But maybe, from up here, I shall be able to see you. Regards, Alan.*'

Now, a man who makes his living evaluating the Hendricks prostates of the world can find it a little difficult to come to terms with the ethereal nature of what I thought I was beginning to understand. I sipped at the whisky and began to read.

An hour later I put the papers down, my mind turning over and over. I thought that I understood, but I could barely begin to grasp the enormity of what I had just been studying so intently.

What lay before me was a meticulously charted, documented and structured analysis of all UFO sightings in Great Britain for the last twenty years. Alan's farm, apparently, stood slap bang in the middle of some ley lines and one of his fields was referred to many times in the papers that now lay at my side.

There were newspaper clippings from all over the world relating to the weird and the wonderful, but with one common theme. Abduction by aliens. The eccentrics, the boffins, the plain crazy – they were all there. And yet there was a simplicity about it that was almost beautiful in its innocence.

I would not, I could not believe it, but clearly Alan did, and I began to feel almost envious of his convictions. But it wasn't true, surely it wasn't true. Was it?

The light was beginning to fade. I don't know how long I had been there but I knew where I had to go. I made my way down to the cornfield with the sun setting and the breeze beginning to rise around me.

All over the cornfield, amongst the gently swaying crop, were large circles of scorched earth with mound upon mound of carefully placed stones, laid out in the precise geometrical patterns of the diagrams in Alan's study. I found that very first one, where I had initially encountered Alan with his arms stretched out to the sky, and looked for the icon.

It was no longer there.

The next few days passed in a blur of police, relatives, work-mates and media attention. Nobody knew, or was admitting to anything. The bank was in turmoil, a major reprogramming project Alan had been involved with apparently having collapsed in his absence. All anyone kept asking me was what did I know, what could I say? Had he been ill, was there another woman, might he have committed suicide . . . ?

And what could I say? 'No, Alan's been abducted by aliens, and he's fine, thanks very much for asking.' It would have been a short trip to a padded cell for me, and I was not in need of that comfort, as yet.

It all settled down after a while. I returned back to normality with the comparative comfort of Mr Hendricks' over-large prostate, the frustrating inability to diagnose Ellen Jenkins' rash and the peculiar bowel habits of the Gresham twins. Every now and then I would drive past the farm, stop, and take a walk in that field, thinking and recollecting. Maggie soon moved away and the farm was sold to people I did not know.

I stopped walking in the field, in the end, but I never stopped remembering.

Two years passed.

Two years of prostates, bowels, rashes and viral infections that didn't need antibiotics but got them anyway because it was easier than arguing. Every now and then I would read an article, or see a programme about UFOs and people who said they had been abducted by aliens, and would smile to myself. They were all crazies, but Alan wasn't crazy. He just believed.

Then one day I received a call from Alan's solicitor, asking me to attend his office. I went with a sense of apprehension and curiosity, sitting reflecting in his waiting room until I was summoned upstairs. He handed me an envelope in silence.

'What's in it?' I asked.

'I haven't a clue,' he replied. 'I was just asked to give it to you two years to the day after he might die, or disappear, and that is what I have done.'

I took the envelope home, but there was no way I could open it there. I drove to the only place I should be and walked out into the cornfield. I sat where the scorched earth had been, took a deep breath, and carefully peeled back the flap.

A note fluttered out in the wind and I scrambled around frantically for a minute or two until I caught it.

It was Alan to a T, typewritten, short, and to the point.

'You always wanted to go to Rio,' it said. 'Please find ten thousand reasons for doing so. The Meridian Hotel used to be good in my day. Regards, Alan.'

I don't know what I expected, really. Well, I suppose I do. I flew to Rio with my wife, half anticipating Alan would be meeting me off the plane, or at the hotel, or just anywhere, yet as the days passed I knew that what I really expected was nothing, nothing at all.

A week after our arrival, my wife having gone sightseeing – in other words shopping – with a newly acquired friend and fellow shopaholic, I sat quietly in a local bar, reflecting and smiling gently to myself.

The barman came across with a glass in his hand.

'Whisky, sir?'

I looked up, surprised. 'I didn't ask for one.'

'No, sir.' The barman pointed to a seat in the corner. 'But he did.'

And there was Alan. Older, greyer, but still the Alan I had known and with the most beautiful – and obviously British – girl at his side, smiling broadly. I walked across, wondering what I thought.

I sat down slowly, my heart beating heavily. We looked at each other in silence for a while, but there was only one thing I could say . . .

'You bastard,' I said, and began to laugh.

Alan threw his head back, grinning hugely, and for the first time I noticed how much weight he had lost. And then I began to understand.

'Hello again, Mike,' he said, wheezing slightly. 'Meet Alana, the one true love of my life.' She smiled at me warmly, holding out her hand.

'Hello, Mike,' she repeated in a low gentle voice. 'I always hoped I might meet you one day.'

'I've been here a week,' I said mildly.

'Just making sure you weren't followed,' grinned Alan wearily. 'I didn't want to be found, not just now.' He drained his drink, motioning for a refill, which came instantly. He saw me notice and winked. 'Oh, money talks in Rio just like everywhere else – although maybe sometimes a little louder.'

He sighed, grimacing in pain, and I could see Alana grimacing with him. 'You want to know why, don't you?'

'Two words, I guess,' I said. 'Malignant, and melanoma. You've got secondaries, haven't you?'

'Still got a few brain cells functioning then. Oh, I knew they were coming, sooner or later. But I've done well, really, nearly two years now since the first of them.' He shrugged in resignation. 'But it comes to us all in the end, doesn't it? I've no more years left now, I'm afraid to say.'

I took another drink, resting my hands on the table. 'It was all just an act, wasn't it?' I said, lighting a cigarette, not knowing how to feel.

He nodded. 'Every single bit of it,' he agreed, shamelessly, 'and God it was fun. You're so respectable, Mike, in an irreverent sort of way. I knew if I could convince you I could convince anyone. I . . . um . . . borrowed a few pounds from the bank and thought I would live a little, before I died. It's been the happiest two years of my life. I have Alana, and well – we have this . . .'

He reached into his pocket, drawing out a photograph of a baby, smiling as babies do, and passed it across. 'Say hello to your namesake, Dr Sparrow. Time to meet Michael Alan Jenkinson.'

We talked for hours that night, and most of the rest of my stay. I saw him for the last time the day before I left to come home.

'Too ill to make it to the airport, these days,' he said, closing his eyes briefly as Alana sat holding his hand. 'Goodbye, Mike. Thanks for everything. We had a lot of fun together, didn't we, you and I?'

I shook his hand one last time, trying not to notice the lump in my throat. 'Yes, we did,' I agreed, looking away quickly. 'Times I will never forget, you bugger you.'

'Hey, write about me when I've gone,' he said as I turned to leave. 'It will be safe, then.'

Every now and then I sit quietly in my study, with the religious icon Alan gave me as we parted, remembering. But always with a smile.

It's not every day that one of your patients is abducted by aliens. And that day, now nearly five years ago, wasn't one of them either.

12

Going Off the Rails

The suicide of a patient brings home the frailty of their life. The suicide of a doctor brings home the frailty of our own. It is a sobering thought.

What made them take their own life? You have the same stresses, the same strains, the same pressures. How can you cope if they did not? And will you?

When a doctor goes off the rails it affects us all.

You never forget your first suicide. Mine, as a GP, was a young farmer who hanged himself from an oak tree on the furthest reaches of his father's estate. He left no note, and nobody ever knew for sure why he had done it. It was hard to know what emotion to feel as I stood there, watching his body sway slowly backwards and forwards in the wind.

All I could think – my senses blunted by the appalling tragedy of the situation – was how did he do it? His father was standing next to me in a state of complete devastation, and I was wondering if he had climbed the tree and thrown himself off, or . . .

I was ashamed of how I felt at the time, but over the years I have learned that shock can bring out the most apparently inappropriate of reactions. We just cope the best we can with whatever we find, trying to rationalise life as we find it. But soon the mind-numbing trauma will pass and you adjust, and move on.

Several years later I was called to a suicide at one of the local residential homes. The patient, a woman in her mid-fifties with a long-standing mental illness, was lying in the undergrowth clutching a framed photo of her recently dead husband in her right hand, the glass cracked and splintered.

By her side lay a bread-knife. She had cut her own throat with one clean stroke, dying instantly. It was a moment both moving and appalling, yet I certified her dead and left, scarcely thinking about it for the rest of the day.

Such are the defence mechanisms we must develop, rightly or wrongly, to survive.

But doctors do not always survive, and their fall from grace can sometimes be spectacular. You only have to recall the case of Clive Froggart, former medical adviser to the Conservative government in the early nineties, who fell prey to the perils of drugs and all they entail.

I have yet to hear the mention of his name in the company of a group of GPs invite anything other than pure contempt or hooted derision, and it may be that he deserves it. It may also of course be because of what he stood for, rather than for who he was.

Perhaps he was a thoroughly nice guy who helped old ladies across the road and did countless unpublicised good works for local charities. But frankly, we did not care.

That was him, and he deserved it, we like to think, but this is us, and we're OK. We haven't degenerated to his level.

Our protection against the thoughts of our own failings and mortality is to deny they may exist, and, by taking comfort in the trials and tribulations of others, we offer them denigration instead of sympathy. It is a road to our own potential ruin, but never will we acknowledge it.

Until maybe it is too late . . .

When I was newly qualified I worked in casualty with a doctor whom I respected tremendously. A year or two older than myself he was, amongst other things, a brilliant musician and widely recognised as being an outstanding physician, destined for great things. Relaxed, knowledgeable and supremely competent, he taught me a tremendous amount in the course of my six-month job.

It is surprising how sometimes you fail to recognise what is staring you in the face. As time passed, I began to realise that two or three times a day he would become pale, sweaty and slightly agitated before disappearing for up to ten minutes at a time.

He would soon return looking more relaxed and confident. Perhaps it was his glasses that prevented me noticing his eyes at first, but then perhaps I just did not want to understand. One day he was absently cleaning his lenses with his tie, a habit of his, and I finally became aware of his pupils, which were highly constricted.

So I asked him.

'Well, you're the first to spot it, Mike,' he said resignedly. ' I knew somebody would, sooner or later. Lucky I held out for so long, I suppose.'

He self-injected diamorphine – heroin, to use its more widely known name – up to six times a day, and had done so for several years. His dose never rose or fell, and he was in control, he said. I believed him, because I liked him and I wanted to. I suppose I was too naïve then to wonder where his supply came from.

He never once asked me not to report him, but I never did. I probably would not if it happened today but I think I would maybe do something else – offer support, or someone else to talk to. But I was too young, too hesitant, too in awe of his experience and professional competence, and besides, I felt it was not for me to judge.

They were his demons and it was for him to deal with them in the best way he could. We lost contact as our jobs came to an end and we each moved on, but I would hear word of him from time to time through the internal network that medicine can provide. And then . . . nothing. He disappeared from sight, and seemed to have gone to ground.

Some years later I was walking through an underpass in London when I heard the haunting refrain of a tune I knew well and stopped, thunderstruck. The musician – long straggly hair, unwashed clothes and the ubiquitous busker's dog – was playing blithely, lost in his music. A few pathetic coppers lay in the hat upturned at his feet. He looked up as I approached and our eyes met. My heart lurched as it was then I knew I knew him; he recognised me too.

He shrugged his shoulders and smiled wryly.

'I lost control, Mike,' he said simply.

In a practice some thirty miles away, in the nearest city, was a GP who had been a close friend of mine at medical school. We had been in the same year, but had lost touch until I moved to the area a couple of years after him.

We met and spoke occasionally, but never somehow rekindled the close friendship of our youth until one day we encountered each other by chance in a pub near my home. The years rolled back in an instant as we sat talking half the night, roaring with laughter at the riotous exploits of the freewheeling days we had shared as students.

He seemed just the same as he was then, and perhaps so did I despite the fact that twenty years had passed in the merest twinkling of an eye. We parted at the end of an enjoyably nostalgic evening, promising to meet again soon.

Three days later he committed suicide, leaving a bemused and devastated wife and two young children. I have no idea why, and his partners have never once spoken of it, either then or now. I just wonder what we might have said to each other that last night in the pub, but somehow never did.

Doctors have one of the highest suicide rates of all the professions. They kill themselves, in part, because they can – it is their final success. A surgeon I once knew dissected out the main arteries in each of his elbows and slit them lengthways – he well

238

knew that if you cut them across they may go into spasm and stop bleeding. I cannot imagine the state of his mind as he did this and to be honest, I do not wish to.

So we have a unique ability to kill ourselves when we reach the point at which we wish to. But what leads us to this stage? If we can understand that, perhaps we can see how we might deal with it.

I do not pretend this is an all-encompassing theory but I offer what I refer to as the 'Baker Effect', which seems to apply most appositely to GPs.

It goes like this . . .

You are a baker, newly qualified and eager to embark upon your chosen profession. You know that you can bake well, and that on average you will need fifty buns a day to offer your customers. You have been working hard at the outset of your career, and already you have several thousand buns in reserve. You are confident that they will last you a lifetime.

You have struggled through your apprenticeship – the long hours, the lack of sleep, the self-doubts – and have survived. Everyone tells you how well you have done, how clever you are, and what a promising future awaits you. You believe every word of it.

At this early stage you have buns for all. Your clients arrive, order their one or two samples each, and are delighted with your services. They find you hard working, obliging and unfailingly courteous. They start by giving you some supplies in return, your stocks rise and you feel wonderful, fulfilled. You want to be able to give them more buns for the same price as just two – three or four each perhaps, so that they feel even better than before.

They are so appreciative of your baking services that they reciprocate, giving you more buns back, maybe even throwing in the occasional doughnut, or a chocolate éclair. Life becomes idyllic, a perfect balance of supply and demand.

Time passes and your reputation spreads. You get more clients, who need more buns, and you start using up your reserves. But still you cannot anticipate a problem – there remain plenty of buns to go round, and you reassure yourself that you can always build up your reserves once more. When you have time . . .

And then your buns begin to go stale, your cakes to crumble. Your customers have been used to three freshly baked items, and now they want four. Then even four becomes no longer enough, and they want five, or even six or seven. You become a victim of your own success, and find it impossible to reduce your services.

If you give them fewer buns, you feel they will stop coming at all. So you start eating your own reserves to give you the energy to bake more. The more you bake, the more they want; the more they want, the harder it is and the more you must eat to keep going. Your reserves are running dry and to preserve the supply to the customers you start looking for another source of food for yourself.

Drink, drugs, affairs . . . broken marriages and short fuses, yet still they need buns. Day after day you are faced with a succession of empty mouths, gnawing away at you like an ever-enlarging nest full of baby birds with a new mouth awaiting you each time you return, exhausted, having to fly further and further for supplies.

They are constantly ravenous and you start looking for a way out, or a means by which you can survive . . .

A colleague in the city fell ill and was off work for a lengthy spell. I knew her well, but was too busy – or, if I could admit it, too thoughtless – to call. It's a sad fact of our lives that GPs are often afraid of other doctors' illnesses, and stay back from close contact. There but for the grace of God . . .

I bumped into her in the library one day, and was staggered by her appearance. I always thought of her as the vivacious, resilient lady in her late thirties that I had known but now she looked near-er fifty, her hair having turned almost completely grey since we last met, and she walked a little unsteadily. I was shocked and must have looked it, and I was guilty and must have looked that, too.

The next week I called at her home to see her – for my sake, or for hers, I wondered for a while – and we began talking. She had three young children, a husband whom she adored but who did not seem able to hold down a job, and a mortgage that seemed to swallow her income.

'I just tried to do too much,' she told me. 'Kids, husband, work, became work, work, kids and husband, and then more work. I just tried to do too much,' she repeated sadly, 'and then one day I found I couldn't do anything at all.' She looked away, tears welling up in her eyes. 'But I had to keep going, somehow.'

I had imagined some chronic debilitating disease, something physical. There was a bottle of gin on the table and she poured herself a large one, pushing one across to me.

'And then there was this,' she said raising her glass in mock salutation, 'but it didn't really help me very much, it just sent me to sleep.'

'I've never known you to drink,' I said aghast.

'No, Mike, you've just never really known me,' she replied quietly. 'But it wasn't even the alcohol, you know . . .'

She rolled up her sleeve and I looked uncomprehendingly at her arm, with its needle marks still harshly visible. 'It was the diamorph,' she added bitterly. 'The wonderful, bloody diamorph.'

Her story came out bit by bit and I listened to the stark details with growing horror. As a young house physician, newly qualified and with the weight of expectation upon her, she was struggling through a long weekend on call with little support. After two consecutive nights without sleep she was all but dead on her feet.

There was only herself and the senior registrar to cope. Worried that she was bound to make a mistake, she went to him in the early hours of Sunday morning to say that she felt she could no longer go on, she was so tired and desperately short of sleep.

'But you have to,' he had told her angrily. 'It's your job. You have to, I have to, all of us have to because everybody expects it of us. It's what we all do for a living.'

The upshot of it was that he gave her some amphetamine to keep her going, and in the depths of fatigue and desperation she took it.

'It made me feel wonderful,' she said with a sigh. 'Oh, so much energy . . . and from then on, when times were bad, I just took whatever was available.'

When general practice became too hard and too demanding, as it does for all of us from time to time, she resorted to what she knew best and what would work. This time I was too sensible, not too naïve, to wonder where her supply came from, and did not need to ask.

It seemed there had been no one to turn to at the time when she needed it most, and being unable to find any support she had struggled along on her own until she could struggle no more. Finally, in desperation, she went to her general practice partner and poured out her troubles to him, pleading for his help.

He had listened in silence and then, as she sat sobbing her heart out in front of him, he picked up his telephone and reported her to the General Medical Council, subsequently banning her from his surgery from that moment onwards. It was as if she had ceased to exist overnight to her patients, and her name was never allowed to be spoken in the practice again.

In truth the reputation of his practice, and ultimately himself, was more important to him than the terrible plight of his partner. In the following weeks he took every step imaginable to distance his name from hers, wasting no opportunity to denigrate her reputation for his own ends.

I wish I could say that this is the only instance I know of a doctor in trouble being deserted by their immediate colleagues, but sadly, it is a far from infrequent occurrence. The perceived opinion of the general public that the medical profession close ranks around each other in times of need is fatally flawed – they do, of course, but only generally to avoid a scandal that may ultimately reflect to a disadvantage upon themselves.

For all that, however, the spectre of Harold Shipman – and, to a lesser extent, the disgraced gynaecologist Richard Neale – casts a shadow across the profession that will not easily be dispersed. So many questions come to mind – how could they do it, for instance? Why did it take so long for anyone to notice, and once they had why were the authorities so slow to take any action?

What is it that makes some doctors believe they are above the law, that the rules will somehow never apply to them? Is it all predetermined? Are we initially attracted to the profession because of some fatal flaw in ourselves, or does the unquestioning faith of so many of those we treat simply turn a few cogs in our heads and make us feel we are that little bit less mortal than those who rely on us to tend to their needs?

Many years ago I worked for a short spell at an air force base where the frailties of the profession were amply demonstrated. None of the following was in itself catastrophic, but who knows where these doctors are today? In your general practice? Awaiting you in outpatients at your local general hospital?

After three years in the RAF I was becoming one of the more senior of the junior GPs, if that makes any sort of sense. As such I was sent to a large station in the north whilst the Senior Medical Officer (SMO) was away on an attachment elsewhere. My remit was to supervise the three junior doctors in his absence.

By the end of the fortnight I was the only one left.

The one female doctor, a spinster of the parish – and probably every other parish she has ever been in since – was now in hospital. After a week of soul searching over some of her increasingly bizarre behaviour I had reported her to the Station Commander as being in my opinion unfit to practise medicine in any capacity. Somewhat to my surprise she had responded by claiming that I was the embodiment of an MI5 plot to get her discredited in the eyes of her patients.

The day following her subsequent interview with the powers-that-be on the station she collapsed with a supposed slipped disc, never to return.

I wonder to this day what became of her.

The youngest doctor, Andrew London, outwardly a pleasant young man, turned out to be spending his coffee breaks regaling the junior members of staff with tales of his supposed sexual exploits as a student. He drove a brand new, glistening white Porsche, a car beyond my wildest dreams in terms of expense – although to be honest I thought it brash and ugly. Give me a beaten-up Morris 1000 any day of the week.

But I always wondered how he managed to finance it, or whether it was even paid for, because he was prey to a whole host of grandiose schemes and ideas. As 'Del boy' he would have been ideal, but as a GP?

Three days after my arrival one of the youngest members of staff, a pretty young aircraftswoman, knocked hesitantly on my door at the end of afternoon surgery.

'Can I talk to you for a moment, sir?' she asked, hovering in the corridor.

'Of course,' I said, gesturing towards a seat. 'It's Sally, isn't it? Come in and sit down. What is it I can do for you?'

'Well, sir . . .' She blushed deeply. 'It's about Flight Lieutenant London . . . I'm not sure I know where to start, sir.'

'Try the beginning,' I said, wondering what was to come.

'Well it's just that . . . I think he . . . he's been asking me to do things, sir,' she blurted out finally. 'Things I don't think I should be having to do. He's been asking me to get things for him.'

She was close to tears.

'Get things?' I asked gently. 'What sort of things do you mean?'

'Off the floor, sir, pick them up for him. He . . . well, he knocks them off the back of his desk and asks me to crawl under it to get them, sir, and I don't know what to do any more . . .'

The other doctor, Jonathan, who was only a year younger than myself, was having an affair with Elaine, the nurse in the medical centre. In civilian life this might not be so unusual, but the nurse was a corporal, a member of the non-commissioned ranks. Relationships between officers and other ranks were strictly forbidden under any circumstances. To make it worse, although Jonathan was single, Elaine happened to be married to another corporal on the same station.

Most of the base, I later came to learn, knew all about it. Most of the base apart from Elaine's husband and the SMO, that is . . .

It was a situation doomed for catastrophe, and inevitably enough catastrophe finally arrived. Late one night Jonathan – who was the duty doctor for the night – came knocking on my door in the officers' mess.

'I just don't know what to do,' he said, pacing up and down my room in a distraught state. 'It's too awful to contemplate . . .'

Elaine's husband, Christopher, had found out that evening about the affair, and taken an overdose. Jonathan, as the doctor on call, had been summoned to treat him . . .

Maybe now they are all out there, well adjusted and fully recovered from the traumas of that evening with their past put firmly behind them. But when you cast a stone into the waters, who knows where the ripples might end?

So how do we approach the inadequacies of our peers? How might they address our own failings? Mostly, I have to say, we do nothing, trusting that somebody else further down the road will take the responsibility from us.

On my last day in a particular job, many years ago, I was in the operating theatre at four o'clock in the morning with the senior registrar. The consultant, Tom MacPherson, was away until lunchtime, but due back to see me on my way before my departure that afternoon.

It was either to wish me well in my future career, to search my luggage to make sure that I was not absconding with any of the hospital property, or simply to make sure that I was actually going, at last.

The patient lying on the operating table before us was an elderly lady who had developed a clot in her femoral artery, the major blood vessel leading down into the leg. She was in great danger of losing both her leg and her life but the registrar had – somewhat to my surprise – clamped the artery above and below the clot with consummate skill, incised the offending vessel and removed the obstruction.

The surgeon was the same Mr Abraham of a previous encounter . . .

Survival was still in the balance, but at least she had a chance. He had all but sewn up the deficit in the artery when he stopped, looking across at me.

'Ever seen a femoral artery bleed, Sparrow?' he asked almost greedily, anticipating the pleasure to come.

I was tired and uninterested. All I wanted to do just then was to finish the case, my morning and my job, before moving on to the next stage of my career.

'No,' I responded shortly. 'And never likely to either.'

'Well, this is your chance, my boy,' he said, and to my horror he released the clamp above his all but completed repair. Fascinated despite myself I watched a great arc of blood curve across the theatre and splatter against the opposite wall, and then again as the next pulse came, and again.

'That's one for your memoirs,' said Mr Abraham, and reached forward to reapply the pressure on the clamp. I can still recall the look of panic dawning across his face as he realised that the clamp had slipped off, and the situation was totally beyond recall.

Feverishly he applied a tight ligature around the artery, closed the wound and snapped, 'Get her out of here. I want her back on the ward before she dies.'

There was silence in the theatre. The skeleton staff just stood, and looked, and wondered.

'She would have died anyway,' he blustered. 'It's just an accident, it happens, it doesn't make any difference to the outcome.' He glared around the room threateningly. 'It's my career on the line here,' he continued harshly, 'and this is one old lady in an out-of-the-way hospital in a nothing town in the north, and nobody will care. And,' he finished menacingly, 'you are all here, all part of this. Now I'm off to get some rest before I have to go to out-patients – clear up here and move her back out to the ward as quickly as you can.'

He stripped off his gloves and his gown, wiped his sweating brow on the back of his sleeve, and departed. The theatre staff all looked at me, and I shrugged. They knew, as did I, that by the end of the day I would be three hundred miles away, but they would be there the next day, and the one after that, having to work with him again, and again, and again . . .

'Do as he says,' I said briefly, 'and leave it to me.'

MacPherson, not entirely to my surprise, failed to turn up as anticipated, and I left without regrets. If he could live without having had the unmissable opportunity to wish me 'All the best' – the universal parting shot of all senior doctors to junior staff whom they had no compunction in ignoring completely from that moment onwards – then so could I. With knobs on.

I wrote to him a week later with a full report of all that had transpired, exonerating the theatre staff completely. My duty done I sat back and waited to be summoned to the GMC for the ensuing case. I waited, and nothing happened, and I waited some more. Then, like all junior doctors, I applied myself to the immediate task in hand and forgot all about it.

The senior registrar later became a consultant and returned to his own country, where I believe he is now a professor. Many years after this happened, when to my eternal discredit I had long since obliterated the original incident from my mind, I met Tom MacPherson's widow by chance when visiting an aged relative in a nursing home in the Midlands.

We talked inconsequentially of various matters, skirting around the subject we both wished to avoid until she fixed me with a piercing stare. Her body may have been failing but her mind was as sharp as a razor, her memory intact to the last detail.

'Go on then, ask me,' she said. 'I know what you're thinking about.'

I hesitated. 'You mean Mr Abraham,' I said at last, 'and my final day in your husband's hospital. I should ask you what happened, what he did in response to my letter. But I already know, don't I?'

She nodded, eyes bright and alert.

'Nothing,' she said. 'Absolutely nothing,' and she nodded again, closing her eyes and leaning back in the chair, remembering. 'He came to me, Tom did, with your letter and asked me what he should do. But we both knew really that what we should, and what we could do, were poles apart.'

She smiled sadly. 'Tom was a good man, but weak. He left Mr Abraham in charge, although we both knew that his behaviour had given everyone cause for concern. We shouldn't have left him but we did. When it was all over on our return it was either his career and possibly Tom's with it, or neither. So it was neither. Expediency above all things. And there had been other cases, cases where they had worked together . . .'

'Mr Prendergast,' I said, remembering, and she nodded.

Mr Prendergast, a man in his early seventies, had come into hospital for investigation into his recent weight loss. It quickly became obvious that he had both a tumour in his rectum, and an unidentified mass in his stomach. Surgery seemed to be his only salvation.

'Which do you want to do first?' I had asked at the end of the ward round.

Abraham and MacPherson looked at each other. 'I think we might try to do them both together,' MacPherson responded. 'I've heard of it being done at other hospitals, and always wanted to have a go. What do you think, Mr Abraham? Shall we give it a go?'

Abraham nodded. 'Be interesting to see how it turns out,' he agreed.

The following day in theatre Mr Prendergast was opened up at each end. His rectal tumour looked to be resectable – in other words removable in one piece, with every hope of a cure – although with some difficulty. MacPherson decided to proceed.

At the same time Abraham had exposed the unidentified mass in Mr Prendergast's stomach, which was smaller than had at first been thought, and stood there looking at it indecisively. In some circumstances surgeons will open up a patient when the precise diagnosis is unclear in order to establish the spread of disease. If it turns out to be significantly greater than expected they may simply close the patient up again without undertaking any other procedures, there being nothing to gain from further intervention.

But there were occasions when you could not be sure, and here there was a standard procedure to be followed. Faced with a lesion which might or might not be cancerous, you took further advice.

'Do you want a frozen section?' I asked.

Normally, when diagnosis was uncertain, a biopsy would be taken. This would then be rushed down to the laboratory for immediate freezing, following which it would be put under the microscope to establish its precise nature. The surgical team meanwhile would just sit and wait in theatre for a telephone call confirming the histology, proceeding on the basis of the result.

'What, and ruin a perfectly good experiment?' said MacPherson, coming round to take a look for himself. 'No, a lump that size has to be malignant. Best take it out whilst we are here.'

Both surgeons continued as previously planned, and Mr Prendergast underwent his two major operations at one and the same time. Two days later, too weak to recover from such extensive surgery, he died. The following day the laboratory reported on the tissue removed from his stomach.

It was benign. His surgery had been unnecessary.

'Yes, Mr Prendergast,' sighed Mrs MacPherson. 'Tom never fully forgave himself for that.'

'Oh poor Tom,' I said bitterly. 'My heart bleeds. But what about me? Did you never think . . . ?'

'Oh, Tom thought about it all the time. He always thought you would come back one day, but I knew what you were like. Young, idealistic, but above all so very busy. Your world had moved on – you would never in a month of Sundays come back to ours. I told him that.'

So justice eluded the unjustified, and we all in our way conspired towards it. Even me – by default, maybe, but that is not sufficient an excuse, it is merely a reason. It seems sometimes that we are all so hell-bent on our own survival, not caring that others may fall, that we dare not risk the failings of others tarnishing our own all-important careers.

The sad consequence of this is that we will not communicate our own fears and inadequacies to our colleagues, lest we be ignored or disowned in return. What would our partners think of us, we fret, they so strong and we so weak and inadequate?

What indeed? The fear of private confession far outweighs the exposure of the public inadequacies.

But maybe our partners and colleagues feel the same. We all have the same problems, we all one day start to run out of buns, we all hover on the brink from time to time . . .

There is no simple answer. I have no more cakes or buns and biscuits than anyone else. But it could be me one day. I might drink more, smoke more and unravel more as well as the rest of them. I just haven't, as yet.

What makes the difference between my friend who committed suicide and myself, or all the others who knew him better?

Maybe he just arrived there first, allowing the rest of us to re-evaluate, to re-establish the priorities in our lives And that is fine, for us, but it doesn't help him, his wife or his children, in any way whatsoever. The suicide of a patient brings home the frailties of their life. The suicide of a doctor brings home the frailty of our own.

13

Mistakes and Misunderstandings

We all of us, whatever our careers or circumstances, make mistakes. Happily they mostly affect ourselves and we alone reap the consequences, but occasionally the effects are projected on to others.

In the world of medicine our mistakes may be simply humorous and harmless, leaving ourselves red-faced and our patients with either fits of the giggles or merely embarrassed sympathy for our inadequacies.

Sometimes, however, our errors may leave a lasting impact on the lives of others, or simply change them for ever.

In the plain silly department, mistaking one patient for another, or confusing their relationships, is something I still do to this day.

We have all done it. Well, I've certainly done it, and I hope to goodness everybody else has, too. A new patient comes into the surgery to register and brings another member of the family with them. You assess their relative ages, and make a calculated decision as to their relationship.

'Well, Mr Thomas,' I recall saying on one occasion, 'you've come down here to live with your mother, have you?' looking at the couple before me. On safe ground here, I thought, he being thirty-two, and his mother fifty-five.

'No,' he replied, straight-faced, 'but I have come down here to live with my wife.'

Exit one doctor stage left, in acute embarrassment.

A young patient of mine in her early twenties came to see me one day, and was obviously struggling to come to the point. I had known her for many years, and had been close friends with her parents who had been tragically killed in a car accident several years earlier.

She had moved away to live with her grandfather, whom I had not met, and only recently returned with him to the area.

'The thing is, Uncle Mike – ' she began.

I raised a hand, and stopped her.

'Tina,' I said gravely, 'I was dangling you on my knee and changing your nappies twenty years ago, and calling me uncle was just fine, then. I could even cope with it when you were a teenager – just.'

She smiled shyly.

'But now you're a grown woman,' I continued, 'calling me uncle just makes me look around for my bathchair and slippers, and pretty soon I shall begin to wonder if I've started dribbling in public and talking to myself whenever I've been alone for more than twenty minutes. So can we drop the "uncle" now, please? For my sake.'

She smiled again, more relieved now. 'OK Unc – OK, Mike. Look, I really came to ask you a favour. I know it's not part of your job, but I just wondered . . . could you as a family friend . . . I mean . . .' She ground to a halt.

'Yes?' I asked encouraging.

'Well, the thing is,' she blurted out after much face pulling and grimacing, 'the fact is, I'm getting married.'

'Tina, that's wonderful,' I said, 'but aren't you . . .' I stopped, just before I got to the patronising part, but she was there before me.

'. . . too young,' she finished for me. 'Don't say it, Mike, we've been through all that, and I'm very happy. The fact is that . . . well, that . . .'

I must have been looking in pre-patronise mode again,

253

because she said slightly irritatedly, 'No, I'm not pregnant.'

'Sorry,' I mouthed.

'He's just a little bit older than me,' she finished lamely.

I considered for a moment.

'A bit?' I ventured non-committally.

'Well – quite a bit,' she said cautiously.

'Could we round it up to the nearest decade, perhaps?'

'Well, you know that I'm nearly twenty-one,' she said carefully.

I nodded.

'Well, he's very nearly . . .' she took a deep breath, 'very nearly sixty-one.'

'That's sort of forty years then,' I worked out quickly.

'I just wondered if you could talk to Grandad for me,' she went on. 'I'm very happy, really, we both are, but Grandad's dead against it.'

We talked for a while longer, and she left reassured after I had agreed to call at their house when I was next passing to do what I could. A few days later, when out on a visit, I realised I was very close to where she and her grandfather were staying and drove the other half-mile to the house.

A fit, bronzed-looking, grey-haired man was sitting in the garden reading a newspaper, and I walked up and introduced myself.

'Hello,' I said, steeling myself for the ordeal to come, 'I'm Dr Sparrow.'

He regarded me steadfastly for a moment, and nodded a greeting. 'I've heard a lot about you,' he said. 'I suppose you've come to talk about Tina. Do you want to go inside?'

'No, here will be fine.' I searched desperately for the right words.

'Now, I know it's difficult for you, and I do understand. I look upon Tina as a sort of surrogate daughter, and I agree, I cannot for the life of me begin to understand why she would wish to marry a man past the age of retirement. It just seems such a waste of her life. But – '

'Perhaps I should stop you right there,' he said, smiling not unkindly.

'I suppose you think it's none of my business,' I began defensively.

'It isn't that.' The corners of his mouth twitched good-humouredly. 'I suppose you think that I'm Tina's grandfather. In fact, he is inside, on the telephone. I've just arrived this morning.'

My heart was already beginning to sink.

'Actually I'm Tina's fiancé,' he continued. 'How do you do?'

Some misunderstandings are just plain silly.

A young man dashed into our reception the other day, shirt half unbuttoned, sweat streaming down his face and in obvious disarray. In a distracted way, strongly reminiscent of a burgeoning White Rabbit, he started muttering, 'I'm late, I'm late. I've got an appointment and I'm late,' and began to explain why.

My receptionist, Christine, scanned the surgery list.

'Are you sure your appointment is today?' she asked. 'I can't find you written down here anywhere.'

'Sure,' he said, flustered, tapping his pockets absent-mindedly. 'I've got an appointment card here somewhere. I'm just late,' and he explained again why.

Christine searched through the list once more. 'I'm sorry, Mr Bus,' she said firmly, 'but you must have the wrong day . . .'

There was silence in reception for a few moments, and then Christine was led away, laughing uncontrollably.

Our reception area is at right angles to the admin office. It was designed that way to stop patients seeing through to where the staff are hard at work, drinking coffee, filing their nails and discussing the previous night's episode of *Coronation Street*. It is also so you can hear them come in but continue to pretend you are busy, thus ignoring them completely for a while, secure in the knowledge that you cannot be overlooked – but it does have its disadvantages.

I was sitting one day at the big grey box in the corner – the rest of the staff call it the computer, but I'm not very technologically minded – when the phone rang.

Christine called across to me, phone in hand.

'Can Mrs Appleby have a word with you, doctor?'

We all have our bad days. 'Not that bloody woman *again*,' I exploded. 'I'm sick and tired – '

I caught the look on Christine's face, and stopped abruptly. Sometimes our staff are just wonderful.

'Not *that* Mrs Appleby,' she said with superb self-control. 'It's the one standing here in reception I'd like you to talk to . . .'

Mostly, when a request for a home visit comes in, I ask for a reason. That way, you know what to take with you, and might even be able to deal with it over the phone. Sometimes, however, if a patient lives reasonably close to the surgery, and rarely calls us out, I will just go and take what I find on spec.

The Wonnacotts were an elderly couple, both hard of hearing, who lived just outside the village. They were devoted to each other. As for many of my patients, life was a constant struggle for them, but they were uncomplaining, happy and rarely troubled us. The surgery was, for once, quiet, and I decided to go right away.

I pulled up at the house, and let myself in. One of the truisms of country practice is that the longer you have been a patient's GP, the less likely you are to knock on the door. Anyway, I knew Mrs Wonnacott was wheelchair-bound and could not negotiate the tiny corridor to the front door, and her husband, despite being in his late eighties, was forever pottering in the garden.

I walked through into the cramped but immaculately tidy living room, where Mrs Wonnacott was sitting with a worried look on her face.

'I'm so sorry to call you, dear,' she began, gently, 'you know I don't like to worry you, but I was a bit concerned about my husband.' She paused.

'Yes,' I said encouragingly, all sorts of ridiculous images flitting through my mind. Gambling, drinking . . . other women. Trainspotting . . .

'Well,' she continued, 'he went out to the wood-shed this morning . . .' It was now four o'clock in the afternoon. '. . . and he hasn't come back. I wouldn't normally call you, but the neighbours are out and I did hope you wouldn't mind.'

My heart went out to her. This poor lady had been sitting in her tiny little house for three hours, unable to get out of the door unaided and worrying herself to death about her husband, before plucking up the courage to ring me for help. I went immediately outside.

The door to the woodshed was slightly open, and inside, I found Mr Wonnacott. He was slumped over his work desk, and was very dead. I gently closed the door behind me, and went back inside.

'I'm so sorry, Mrs Wonnacott,' I said, sitting down beside her, 'but I've found your husband in the woodshed, and I'm afraid I have to tell you that he's dead.'

'Oh yes, I know that, dear,' she responded, completely unconcerned. 'Where did you say he was again?'

'In the woodshed,' I said, raising my voice slightly and feeling rather out of control of the situation.

She patted me on the hand. 'I'm sorry to bother you again, dear, when you've already been so kind. But would you mind asking him to come in? He's already missed his lunch, and it's nearly time for tea.'

Shock, I thought. It hadn't set in, she would not accept it. To be left alone after all those years together – it was just too much for her to bear.

'Mrs Wonnacott,' I said a little more loudly, 'I'm afraid that your husband is dead.'

She squinted up at me, looking a little exasperated.

'Yes, dear, I do know that, I already told you. He's been deaf for years.'

OK, so I smoke.

Yes, I know it means a hideous death in searing pain, or a tortuously slow, lingering demise in abject misery and suffering at the taxpayer's expense.

But I *like* to smoke, for goodness sake.

The attitude of us smoking GPs to those patients who smoke is perhaps unsurprisingly more tolerant than that of our brethren who pride themselves on being purer in heart and spirit. We do not treat them as being akin to Attila the Hun, or Hitler's nastier brother, but welcome them as fellow human beings, flawed but all the more interesting for their failings. And besides, we can always borrow a light from them in an emergency.

So when I was given a message by one of our receptionists that the nursing home had rung to say that dear old Reg Harris was chain-smoking and was that all right, I thought – of course it was. The poor old chap was terminal with presumed – though unproven – carcinoma of the bronchus (lung cancer) and deserved in my opinion any little pleasures he had left. OK, he was on continuous oxygen, but at least if he blew up the east wing of the nursing home he would go out with a bang and earn a footnote in the local press for his trouble.

'Give him my blessing,' I said, 'and leave him be.'

We had at that time a medical student with us in the practice who was now into her second week of discovering all the very good reasons we could think of for not becoming a GP. She had seemed almost normal on her arrival – or as normal as anyone can be who is still bent upon a medical career – keen, interested, enthusiastic and knowledgeable, and quite unlike her temporary mentor.

A middle-aged farm worker sat before us, and I had given him my normal intensely personal individual greeting ('What can I do for you, Mr Jones?') as opposed to 'What can I do for you, Mrs Smith?' or 'What can I do for you, Reverend Jenkins' – you get the picture.

'I've got a pain in me guts,' he had said. Cue immediate loss of interest from GP, cunningly concealed as a generous attempt to give our student a gift-wrapped opportunity to explore her burgeoning medical knowledge.

'Would you like to ask Mr Jones a few questions about his pain, Nikki?' I asked, thinking this might be an ideal opportunity to slip out for a quiet fag and a coffee.

Think again. Nikki's face had become suffused with a worryingly reddish hue, and she was visibly shaking with an emotion I was unable to immediately identify.

'Nikki?' I asked again.

'I can't . . . think of any,' she said, waving a hand weakly in submission. She was still breathing, I noticed, so I gave up. Sadly, I had to deal with the patient myself, and wait another five minutes for my nicotine/caffeine fix.

The day passed without further undue incident, and as we were poised to leave that evening I suddenly recalled Nikki's rather odd behaviour of that morning.

'Oh, that,' she said, blushing an interesting vermilion colour. 'I thought he said, "I've got a pain in me nuts!" and it just threw me completely.' She collapsed in helplessly silent giggles and I was just thinking about joining her when my earlier phone call sprang into my mind.

I ran to my car, dragged open the door and drove off as fast as I could down the road. Sometimes misunderstandings are just plain funny whereas others . . . I pulled up at the door of the nursing home, charged up the stairs three at a time (well, two and then one, to be honest – it was three storeys, and I do smoke too much) and burst over-exuberantly into poor old Reg Harris's room about two minutes before he died.

Some years probably before I was born, a Dr Stokes and a Dr Cheyne produced the definitive study of the interrupted, sighing breathing pattern patients often develop shortly before they die. They gave it their name, and it lives on today.

He wasn't chain-smoking. He'd given up ten or more years ago. He was Cheyne Stoking . . .

Of course, patients make mistakes too, and these happy events are most enjoyable of all when they make mistakes with each other and leave you out of it altogether.

One thing you must never do is laugh outright at a patient's predicament. Particularly if they are still in the room at the time. Of course, some medical schools prepare you for this arduous forthcoming trial of self-restraint by telling you the five funniest jokes known to man at your interview. Maintain a stony, silence throughout, and you're in.

Before me now sat Norman Prescott, a kindly, good-humoured chap in his mid-forties, with a slightly quizzical look on his face as if he could not quite understand how he came to be here at all. His right arm was fully plastered courtesy of a fractured humerus, and he winced occasionally as a spasm of pain shot through his broken (in two places) collar bone. He was not normally given to athletic or dangerous pursuits, and I asked him how this had happened.

'Well, it was a lovely day on Sunday,' he said good-humouredly, 'so I thought I would cut the lawn, and catch some sun at the same time. Shorts, sandals, sun hat and off I went. I said hello to my next-door neighbour over the fence, Colin Westlake – you know him, don't you . . .'

I nodded, intrigued. Colin was an amiable giant of a man, good-hearted but stronger in the brawn than the brain department.

'. . . who was digging his vegetable patch. I've got one of those old electric mowers – very good, but it's a swine to restart if you let it stop. Anyway, as I was cutting away, I got a stone in my sandal. Fortunately I was just by the fence and didn't want to stop, so I leant against it and started to try and shake the stone out.'

I felt this bubbling sensation in my stomach beginning to rise, as I sensed an uncontrollable moment ahead.

'You can see what's coming, can't you?' continued Norman, ruefully shaking his head. I could. I couldn't speak, and nodded weakly.

'Colin, next door, saw me holding my electric lawn mower, leaning against the fence and shaking vigorously. He thought I was having an electric shock and knew he would have to do something fast . . .'

I was openly crying now.

'. . . so he did. He ran up to the fence, raised his arms and hit me with his spade across my right shoulder to make me let go.'

You must never ever laugh at a patient's misfortune. It's just that sometimes it is impossible not to.

It's strange how some things seem to become a recurring image of general practice. Death, babies . . . and false teeth, for instance.

A patient of mine, Emily, a young girl I had known since her pre-teen days, recently took up her first job in one of the social service-run residential homes. I have no experience of them – at least, none I am admitting to – but on my rare visits there it always reminded me of a soup kitchen for the socially deprived.

She came to me one day in a state of some distress, having just started her first spell of night duty. Tears were welling in her eyes as she began to talk, twisting her handkerchief round and round in her hands, as if it somehow held the answer to all her problems if only she could just wring it out hard enough.

'I wanted so much to be a success,' she said with a catch in her voice. 'I know it's not the grandest job in the world, but it's so difficult to find work around here and it really meant something to me.'

It was impossible not to feel for her.

'Then you've lost your job?' I asked.

She shook her head repeatedly. 'No, it's not that.' Her voice tapered away. 'I just feel so stupid,' she whispered finally.

One of her duties in her first night's work was the 'False Teeth' round. Apparently, although the elderly residents were generally quite good at removing their teeth by night, they were less good at washing them thoroughly before returning them whence they came the following morning. It was Emily's task, room by room, to wash their teeth as they slept.

'They gave me this big bottle of disinfectant stuff and told me to wash and dry every set. There were so many of them, I was worried I wouldn't get round, and they're always so short-staffed there, so I thought I'd find a better way of doing it.'

All right so far, I was thinking. Showing initiative, time management skills . . . where's the problem?

'So I collected all the teeth, took them down to the kitchen, washed them all together in the soup vat, and put them to dry in the oven.'

I tried not to chuckle, as a vision of row after row of false teeth baking quietly next to the hot cross buns came into my mind.

'It was so much quicker,' she said, allowing herself a small wry smile. 'It took only half the time it normally does . . .' Her voice tailed away again.

'And?' I prompted encouragingly. 'What was wrong with that, Emily?'

She burst into uncontrollable floods of tears, and I silently pushed across the box of tissues on my desk. She clutched a handful gratefully, and her sobs slowly subsided.

'Trouble was,' she said, 'when it was all done I had eighty-five sets of false teeth and I didn't know which pair belonged to which resident.'

And while we are on the subject of false teeth . . .

One of the prerequisites for a successful career in medicine is the ability to remain completely straight-faced and unperturbed in the presence of a patient when the awful truth dawns upon you of the unimaginable howler you have just committed.

The nurse in this story deserves to go far.

Death on a hospital ward is always followed by a slightly surreal ritual. The recently departed is laid out according to local protocol, duly certified as being no longer in need of canteen services, and then prepared for transfer to the mortuary.

In the country there are still ladies in many villages who perform the duties of 'laying out' by time-honoured tradition – their mother did it, and their grandmother before them. You see them, pedalling out in their Sunday best on a Thursday and neighbours nodding sagely together, 'Mabel's off to do her duties. That'll be old Mr Bowers gone, then.'

The main aim in a hospital is to conceal the death of the patient from all the others on the ward, to avoid adversely affecting their own recovery by witnessing the demise of one of their erstwhile colleagues.

To this end, all the curtains are drawn around the other beds to prevent their occupants witnessing the mobile coffin being wheeled on to the ward, duly filled with the late departed, and wheeled out again.

The simple fact is, of course, that you can always hear the wretched thing being wheeled in. They have an unmistakable clankety sound. Besides, the only time the curtains are ever all drawn on the ward apart from night time is when somebody has died and they want to get rid of the evidence, thus immediately drawing everybody's attention to the precise fact they are trying to conceal.

I am sure the protocols should be rewritten. In my version, as soon as a death is observed (hopefully, but not always, within twenty four hours of the event itself) the two largest and jolliest nurses on the ward would be dispatched with a wheelchair – in full, unobstructed view of the rest of the ward – to the bed in question.

'Come on, Mr Tomlinson. Time for your daily constitutional. My, are we sleepy today – bit of a late night last night? Come on now, no answering back. You are a one . . .'

They would then load the late Mr Tomlinson into the wheelchair, sit him bolt upright – maintaining his position with judiciously placed sticky tape, if necessary (all in a good cause) – and propel him down the ward in full view of all those present. I swear that no one would take a scrap of notice.

The 'Mr Tomlinson' in this particular case had been duly deposited in the mortuary when the young nurse who had taken him there returned to his bed to change the sheets for some freshly laundered ones. An older nurse, of course, ever conscious of the pressing financial restraints of our glorious health service, would have improvised and merely swapped them with the sheets on the nearest available empty bed.

With sudden horror, having drawn back the curtains, she noticed that his false teeth had been left on the cabinet by the side of his bed. Full of concern, she slipped them quickly into the pocket of her uniform, thankfully observing the unoccupied bed next door. No one had spotted the mistake.

'I felt so awful,' she told me later. 'I should have noticed. Poor man, him being taken away without his teeth, it's just so undignified. So I rushed down to mortuary – the ward thankfully was quiet for a few moments – pulled back his sheets and put his teeth back in for him. It was a bit of a struggle, but then I've never had to put a pair of false teeth back into a corpse before and eventually I managed it.'

She then dashed back to the ward, feeling part flustered, part exhilarated at having succeeded, and saw the occupant of the bed next to 'Mr Tomlinson' now returned and waving her across to him.

He's going to ask me about Mr Tomlinson, she thought worriedly. He'll be so upset. What am I going to say?

She walked slowly across to the foot of his bed, smoothing her uniform down as she went.

'I've just been for a bath, nurse,' said the ruddy-faced man belligerently, 'and when I got back, well, I can tell you, I had a bit of a shock.'

'I do understand your sense of loss,' she said soothingly, 'we all do. But these things happen, I'm afraid.'

He stared at her uncomprehendingly. 'I've no idea what you're wittering on about,' he said, 'all I want to know is, where's me false teeth? I left them right here on the locker . . .'

Training counts. Without a flicker of an eyelid she said calmly, 'Saw they were there, Mr Johnstone, thought we'd give them a bit of a clean. All part of the service. Should be ready in the next few minutes.'

She rushed back to the mortuary, prised the teeth out of the late Mr Tomlinson – 'Harder to get them out than to put them in,' she told me later, 'rigor mortis having set in, just a bit' – and returned them to their rightful owner.

'There, Mr Johnstone,' she said brightly. 'You wouldn't believe how much trouble we've been to.'

Mrs Ellery Dawe is a venerable lady in her late eighties, with a stern eye and razor sharp mind, who after some fifty years' abstinence from the surgery – not to mention a little more abstinence from some other less exciting pastimes – came in to see me one day bringing with her a prolapse I swear she must have been nurturing for a good twenty years.

'Last three doctors I saw were at the hunt,' she said by way of introduction, 'and all of 'em dead, now. Do you hunt, young man?'

The only thing I know about horses is that sitting on one hurts almost as much as one of them sitting on you, and that both eventualities are to be avoided at all costs. However, I did not want to disappoint her too much, partly through my natural politeness and partly through abject fear. She terrified me.

'Not all that often,' I replied lamely, 'not as often as I would like. Pressure of work, family, that sort of thing.'

'Ever?' she asked firmly, fixing me with that gimlet eye.

I crumbled. 'Never,' I admitted, crushed.

'Thought so,' she said, slapping her thigh with an imaginary riding crop whilst I ducked inadvertently.

For the purposes of this brief anecdote I must explain that I have two children, Charles and Cressida, whom I adore equally and unreservedly, and in whose hands I am abject putty. My son, bless him, does not yet realise how intelligent he is, and has a decent underlying goodness and humanitarianism that I cannot for one moment believe is genetically predetermined.

And there is my daughter – at the time of writing aged nine – who was once looked after by our practice counsellor when I was caught in a late surgery.

'Parliament or Parkhurst,' she told me afterwards. 'Definitely one of the two.' I am not at all sure which of those I would prefer for her, come to think of it.

'Do you shoot?' asked Mrs Dawe, looking for some redeeming feature. 'Pheasant, I mean.'

'No,' I admitted. 'I miss them on purpose.'

She spent a few moments trying to decide if this was a joke or not, before continuing, 'Fish?'

'Er, no.'

'Go to the Countryman's' – a local haunt of the hunting/shooting/fishing fraternity – 'on Wednesdays or Fridays?'

'No.'

'Good,' she said briskly. 'Then we are never likely to meet in a social capacity. You may now examine my prolapse, young man, and treat my thrush.'

'Thanks,' I said, with just a hint of gentle sarcasm, but it went happily wide of the mark. She did indeed have a prolapse – and one to be proud of – as well as vaginal thrush (a common enough complaint in women, known medically as candida), and I explained this to her and treated her for it. The prolapse – and its owner – I referred to one of the local gynaecologists.

Mrs Dawe, incidentally, confirmed par excellence one of my theories regarding hysterectomies, that the younger you are when you part company with your womb, the longer it takes you to recover. Three weeks after her operation I called to visit and found her lugging a sack of coal from the garden shed, not generally part of the recommended recovery package.

'Never felt better,' she responded forcefully when I ventured to scold her for her unwarranted activity. 'Can't see what all the fuss is about. It was more out than in anyway.'

But back to that first consultation. Just when I thought I had weathered the storm she fixed me with an eagle eye and said:

'Tell me, young man. Why did you name your daughter after a vaginal complaint . . . ?'

This is almost a complete non sequitur, and of no relevance to general practice itself save for the chronology, but half-way home from surgery that lunchtime I passed a patient of mine out walking his Dobermann. My publisher, on reading this the first time, dismissed it as being an 'urban myth', but I can assure you that it really happened.

I am by no means a vet, and have never wished to be – wherever my right arm may one day find itself, never have I had the desire for it to be fully inserted in a cow's rectum at three o'clock in the morning in an unheated barn on the outskirts of Dartmoor, looking for something I had no real wish to discover – but there was no doubt the dog was not well. My patient, recognising my car, was flagging me down vigorously.

I stopped and slowly disembarked, wishing he had a predilection for Yorkshire terriers, or even Chihuahuas. The Dobermann was coughing and retching, gasping for breath, and seemed happily uninterested in that soft vulnerable area between my head and my shoulders.

I was confident I would live, which was quite enough for me, but of the Dobermann I was less sure. I bundled my patient and his dog into my car – hoping fervently none of us would be sick within the next ten minutes – and, with a great sigh of relief (having counted all four of my limbs and found them still present), dropped them both off at the vet's as we pulled into the village.

I thought no more of it for a couple of days – after all, what's an ailing Dobermann when you have Antonia Bentley's constipation to consider, not to mention her son's curious habit of . . . well, I should probably draw a veil over that, save to mention the word 'hamster' in hushed tones – and then I bumped into my patient in the post office.

'Oh, he's fine, thanks,' he said, in response to my inquiry. 'The vet looked in his throat and said, "I think you'd better go home now," and I asked him why. "Well, somewhere near you there's a hand with two fingers missing," he answered, "and I think I've just found them."'

'So I called in at Geoff's' (the local policeman) 'on the way, and we both went back to my house. There, in the conservatory, was an unconscious burglar lying in a pool of blood with two of his fingers missing . . .'

Our phone number is similar to the vet's and we frequently get calls intended for them.

'Popsy's got piles,' you might hear – a perfectly normal daily complaint. 'Can you give her something for it over the phone, or do I need to bring her in?'

'Yes, of course,' our receptionist might say. 'Has she had this problem before?'

'A couple of months ago, and the cream worked splendidly. Oh, and can I have some more of those charcoal dog biscuits?'

I received a phone call one day from a very agitated farmer's wife, a recently registered patient that I had not as yet met.

'Please, please hurry,' she gasped. 'It's my baby. I think she's swallowed a piece of wire, and she's choking.'

I took some directions, and promised I would be there as quickly as I could. It is a truism of country life that GPs drive down the winding hedge-bordered lanes like sales reps on the motorway, except that sales reps have been known to use their brakes occasionally. I once raced through our village (speed limit 30 mph) at something over ninety miles an hour, only to encounter the village policeman standing by his patrol car at the local garage. His response was typical – no wagging finger, no speed camera at the ready, and no notebook flipped open in his hand to take my number. He just crouched down by his car, cradling his head in his arms in mock horror, and grinned as I whizzed past.

I drove to the farm as fast as I could, all sorts of possibilities passing through my mind. Would the baby still be alive? Would I have to do my first emergency tracheotomy on an infant? Would there be any chocolate biscuits left in the coffee room by the time I returned?

I screeched to a halt in the farmyard and breathlessly ran into the kitchen.

'Where is she?' I panted. 'How is she? How old is she?'

The farmer's wife, a plump, red-cheeked lady in her early forties, grasped my hand in appreciation.

'Oh, you're new to the area, aren't you?' she sobbed.

'Well, I was ten years ago,' I murmured politely.

'But thank you so much for coming,' she continued. 'She's this way.' She waddled across the courtyard and into a dilapidated barn.

Strange place for a baby, I thought.

'Over there,' motioned my hostess, 'in the corner.'

I moved forward, in some trepidation, and encountered my patient. Our eyes met, and we regarded each other with some interest.

'Mrs Holsworth,' I said slowly, 'I feel I have to tell you something.'

'Can't you do anything?' she pleaded. 'I do love her so, please help if you can. Don't tell me she's going to die.'

'It's not that, Mrs Holsworth.' I was struggling for words. 'It's just that I'm not actually the vet . . . but this is an ostrich!'

I have also treated a Jack Russell with heart failure, undertaken a pregnancy test on a horse, and once inadvertently sent my district nurse to perform an enema on a Vietnamese Pot-Bellied Pig. I don't know which of us was more surprised – she, myself, or the pig – when she achieved her objective. I even once treated five hundred hamsters with a stomach bug . . .

There was one occasion when a man barged into my surgery late one evening, thrust his jaw truculently towards me and rested his knuckles on my desk like an orang-utan auditioning for a part in a Clint Eastwood film. I formed the impression he might be a trifle upset.

'You there!' he expostulated at full volume. 'Tell me, are you having an affair with my wife?'

I had never seen this chap before in my life, and decided I would not be unduly perturbed should we never meet again. He was unquestionably larger and angrier than myself, and looked as if he had been badly hewn from a lump of granite by an apprentice sculptor with a drink problem.

A number of exquisitely diplomatic responses raced through my mind. Like, 'Not at the moment,' or, 'Why, is she offering?' and even 'Give me a chance to finish evening surgery first.'

I quickly put such flippancy far from my mind. The man needed appeasing, and fast. I considered my response carefully, and after due thought resolved to be completely serious.

But I failed. 'I don't know,' I responded truthfully. 'What does she look like?'

My practice is based in a fairly isolated village, encompassing several equally isolated satellite villages and small hamlets. Public transport is all but non-existent, and many of our patients are either elderly or of insufficient means to possess their own car.

When it comes to ordering repeat prescriptions, we improvise. We leave them at post offices, village shops and next-door neighbours. We utilise – on occasion – the postman, the newspaper boy and the milk-lady. It is probably clinically completely unsound, but it is both practical and realistic.

Our receptionists tend to live in outlying areas as well, so we use them too.

I called at one of our branch surgeries, my normal Thursday morning routine, and took the orders for my return back to base. Once there, I smiled sweetly at my receptionist, employing all the usual emotional blackmail techniques – 'so old, so in need, and not so far out of your way' – and following it up, as usual, with the hollow promise of a pay rise, and gave her the two packets to deliver.

It had been business as usual. Young Sarah, who had recently delivered a first and long-awaited bouncing baby boy, had piles. Ethel Barriball had a chest infection. Their respective medication once prepared, our new receptionist, Joan, promised to drop the packets in on the way home, and I erased it from my mind.

A few days later, the phone rang and the call was passed through to me. It was Sarah.

'How's that new young man of yours?' I asked. 'Any problems?'

'Oh no, doctor,' she explained, 'everything's fine. Jamie's brilliant, and so good. It's just about my suppositories – I meant to ring you the other day. It's just that with a new baby and all I haven't got around to it.'

'Yes, Sarah,' I replied absently. 'What's the problem?'

'Well, somebody very kindly put the prescription through my door . . .'

'Yes?'

'But it looks like antibiotics, to me. Has there been some sort of mistake?'

Sarah and Mrs Barriball lived next door to each other. My receptionist had inadvertently put the wrong packet through the wrong door. A simple mistake, and so easy to understand.

But the worrying thing was that Ethel had never noticed. I just wondered what she had done with the suppositories . . .

Some misunderstandings are so pathetically stupid that you wonder how you can ever hold your head up in public again without resorting to a balaclava worn in reverse.

When I joined the RAF, I was sent to be a GP for a year at an outlying station. I had no training, experience, competence or to be frank, ability, but no one seemed to be unduly concerned. Apart from me.

I arrived on a Sunday afternoon, and wandered along to the medical centre where the staff were holding a relaxed barbecue. I looked at my boss in waiting, and his wife and three children, a picture of domestic bliss, and thought how old and boring he seemed. I was then twenty-five, and he thirty-two.

Oh, the callowness of youth.

I knew little then of general practice, or of GPs, save that I had nothing in common with my fellow professionals and that they all became terminally boring by the age of thirty. All that has changed, of course. It actually takes until about the age of fifty, but I reserve the right to re-amend in about ten years from now.

I approached my first morning in the job with some trepidation.

I had in my previous year helped amputate limbs, strolled the corridors of the intensive care unit with confidence, inserted scalpels into a wide variety of abdomens, and, most dangerous of all, attended nurses parties without a chaperone. I was well bloodied in the traumas of emergency medicine.

But deal with a teenager's acne? Recognise a case of measles? Talk to old-age pensioners about their loss of libido? Quite frankly, I did not have a clue. I was very relieved, therefore, when my first patient, a young Welsh airman, came straight to the point.

'Think I've got a problem with my urine,' he said in his lilting accent. 'Like you to test it, sir, if you would.'

I breathed a sigh of relief. Simple, wasn't it?

'Does it smell?' I asked.

He looked at me in disbelief. 'My urine?'

'Yes,' I said. Poor chap was obviously a bit slow. 'Is it cloudy? Any blood in it? Do you have to get up at night?'

'Are you winding me up?' he asked, adding a quick, 'sir,' as an afterthought.

'Not at all,' I replied honestly. 'I'm just trying to find out a bit more about it.'

'I don't know what you're on about, sir. I just want you to test my urine.'

I sighed, and reached behind me for a urine pot.

'Put some of it in there,' I said, 'and bring it back to me when you've done.'

He looked frankly bewildered, then cross, and then rather pitying.

'I've got a problem with my urine,' he said slowly.

'Yes,' I agreed.

'My uring,' he repeated, sticking a forefinger in each ear. 'My *uring* . . . H, E, A, R, I, N, G. Uring.'

I never could quite get to grips with the Welsh accent. I hid beneath my desk for the rest of the morning.

14

Night Visits and Alsatians

Night visits are the bane of a GP's life. Along, that is, with day visits, weekends on call, telephone calls, paperwork and, in fact, the patients themselves, come to think of it.

But night visits rule.

It is a concept that somehow seems to elude the sensitivities of our patients. They spend a restless night with a sick relative, and become tired and irritable. We work all day, go out on night visits, work all the next day, go out on night visits . . . and we become tired and irritable too.

And yet, though it seems entirely appropriate for a patient to be irritable with his doctor, the converse is apparently unacceptable. One of life's great unsolved conundrums, to be sure.

Anyway, back to night visits. I think they provide the single most wide-ranging set of emotions of any of our duties. Let me explain.

It is three thirty in the morning, and boy, is it cold outside. But I am warm, comfortable and asleep, dreaming of . . . well, never mind what I am dreaming of. We start therefore in a state of bliss, until the phone rings.

I hope it is for the wife. Strange how it always turns out to be wishful thinking. I realise that I'm no longer married – relief – and that it must be for me – resignation. I answer it – irritation – and it's a wrong number – delight. I go back to sleep – bliss again – until the phone rings once more at three forty-five.

It's Mrs Beckett – horror – and her youngest child is screaming in the background – distaste.

I try to think of every excuse I can not to leave the sanctuary of my bed, only partly because I saw Mrs Beckett's second youngest child screaming at three forty-five yesterday morning and the novelty begins to wear thin. The other part is fatigue, disinclination and abject misery, in equal measures.

I resign myself to driving through the night – dreariness. The heater isn't working again – despair – and eventually I arrive at my destination, shivering with cold. I traverse the unlit drive hoping fervently I can avoid the copious amounts of animal excrement I know lie all around me – distaste and reluctance again.

Distaste lingers through this entire visit, come to think of it, occupying pole position for much of the time.

I enter the house. Mrs Beckett's youngest is now fast asleep and she refuses to let me wake him up – distaste again, but tempered with silent relief. At least I won't have to touch him, this time – he is always grubby, smelly and in need of a new nappy – nausea, and lots of it.

I leave, and in my excitement at being let off so lightly I am less careful where I tread. Nausea becomes the dominant sensation on the journey home, with distaste a very strong second. I climb into bed, falling asleep quickly, and life is blissful once more.

Until the phone rings again . . .

It's a pretty negative mix, when you consider it. And the moral of this tale?

All GPs should sleep more and consider divorce. It gives us the most positive emotions of our lives.

All visits can be unpredictable, but night visits are in a class of their own.

As you and I may lie awake in the early hours worrying about one of the major traumas in our lives, like how *could* West Ham lose in the third round of the FA Cup to Swansea, for goodness sake, there are other people out there worrying about their health.

Why don't they worry about mine, for a change?

But no – are they losing weight, they wonder? Will they still be constipated tomorrow? Can you really get piles from sitting on cold radiators and for how long do you have to do it?   A patient of mine once said – and I swear this is true – 'I sat on a cold radiator for twenty minutes once after the war. Do you think that might have done it?'

'No, Mrs Jordan,' I replied with a sigh. 'I think it a little unlikely.'

'Must have been that last pregnancy of mine, then,' she said reflectively.

'Or the other thirteen before it,' I muttered viciously, snapping on my plastic gloves and reaching malevolently for the lubricating cream.

'This will probably hurt,' I added, 'but do look on the bright side. It's only four o'clock in the morning, the night is yet young and it won't hurt me anywhere near as much as it's going to hurt you . . .'

I was once called out on a beautiful moonlit night by a patient who would only tell me on the telephone that he was worried, but couldn't bring himself to explain why. So why did you go, I hear you cry, and I can't think of a good answer to that save for the fact I was young, idealistic, his niece was staying with him at the time and I had a bet with my partner that I would get her in a bedroom before him.

The sheer unadulterated pleasure of seeing her answer the door in the flimsiest of nightdresses (she was a patient of another practice, by the way, and it is perfectly acceptable to lust after those) was somehow lost in the subsequent banality of the call.

Mr Quilly was sitting up in bed, a perturbed expression on his aged and wrinkled face. 'Thank you so much for coming, doctor,' he said, beaming up at me. 'I'm sure you can put my mind at rest. Tell me, why *is* it that my left foot smells so much more than my right?'

As I have previously mentioned, I used to be in the RAF. Well, somebody had to. I was doing an obstetrics job, working all day and every other night (babies, incidentally, are always, *always* born less than half an hour after you have finally gone to sleep), and on my nights off I would moonlight, covering for the local GPs.

It doesn't make for sanity – or what remains of it after four years as a junior hospital doctor – but it doesn't half help pay the mortgage.

I had been out on three calls that evening, becoming progressively colder each time, and had fallen asleep probably fractionally before opening my front door. I don't remember clambering into bed, but I certainly remember waking up, telephone in hand.

'Issa denabas,' a voice was bellowing in my ear. 'Issa denabas.'

Now, I don't pretend to be the world's most knowledgeable doctor, but I was pretty sure that the 'denabas' was a disease rarely encountered by mankind to date. I had, in fact, never heard of it.

'What are the denabas?' I tried.

'Issa denabas,' he repeated stubbornly.

'Could you be a bit more specific?' I suggested.

'Issa denabas,' he persisted.

'Can you tell me a little more about it?' I ventured.

'Issa denabas,' he reiterated.

Ten minutes later, I knew the denabas did not hurt and were not actively bleeding, but was otherwise none the wiser. My mood – not to mention my wife trying in vain to sleep beside me – had become increasingly agitated and I had reached, I thought, my point of maximum frustration. But not quite.

Reluctantly, I decided to visit. It would be quicker to drive into town and back than to try and elicit any further positive information over the telephone.

'Where do you live?' I asked.

'Nexta da garage,' he said, and put the phone down.

There were precisely forty-three garages in Swindon.

Forty-two garages later, I actually found the house. It had to be the one, as every single other occupant of Swindon was asleep, save for me, and this house had a light on. I knocked on the door, which swung slowly open in front of me.

I stepped tentatively inside.

A dimly lit room met my eyes, and gradually, as my sight adjusted to the gloom, I could see all around me. What I could not see, however, was my patient.

The door creaked shut behind me. I have never been summoned to a haunted house, but just at that moment, as the door swung eerily in the silence with the embers of the fire glowing gently in the grate, I felt that experience would no longer be necessary.

And then the spell was broken.

An emphysematous cough rumbled towards me, and I turned with a start to see a small and wizened Polish man (no, I am not psychic, I learned he was Polish later in the consultation) standing before me, his back to the door and brandishing an equally wizened walking stick just inches from my nose.

'Issa denabas,' he muttered, waving his stick in the general direction of the fireplace.

I cannot recall the precise conversation that followed. My memory has blanked out the greater part of it, and I am very grateful for that too. What I do remember is that some ten surreal minutes later, when it was even money as to which of us would hit the other one first – bearing in mind he would merely have lost his walking stick had he done so, I quite possibly my career – I said very slowly and deliberately, 'Tell me what the denabas are now, or I leave and you may possibly die from them.'

He all but spat at me in his frustration, and then relinquished his guardianship of my exit, staggered across to the fireplace and smote the wall beside it with surprising ferocity for one so small. A short blast of loud music burst forth from the house next door.

'Issa da nabas!' he shouted.

There are times in all our careers when we truly wonder why we bother, and this was the point when I wondered if I could ever bother again. It was not the denabas. It was da nabas. It was the *neighbours*, the bloody neighbours . . .

Apparently, the neighbours had had a late night party and kept him awake with music of a not entirely quiet and harmonious nature. He had, it transpired, called the police, the fire brigade, the Red Cross – no, I don't know why, either – ambulance control and the emergency social services to complain, and they had all politely declined to attend. So he had called me.

I was the only one apparently stupid enough to respond. I felt that positive action was called for, so I strode across to the fireplace, banged as hard as I could on the wall with my fist and shouted in my best (in fact, only) Polish accent, 'Turna da bloodya musica downa. How manya more timesa?'

And then I left, being rewarded, as I got wearily into my car, by the body-wrenching beat of rekindled music from next door splitting the silence of the night. The Rolling Stones. 'Sympathy For The Devil.'

Half-way home, I started laughing.

Widemouth Bay, on the Devon/Cornwall border.

It is four o'clock in the morning, and a vicious winter night out. We have been driving for three-quarters of an hour and seen no cars, no lights, no sign of life anywhere in the vicinity. No one with any sense would be out on a night like this. But my driver and I are.

After years of working punishing out-of-hours rotas – every other night, every other weekend on call, not forgetting the day job – life had suddenly changed, with my partner and I rejoining the human race.

The debilitating effect of consistent night duty in addition to the daily grind creeps up on you in due course. You become shackled to the telephone, unable to relax, just waiting for that next call. Fatigue is an omnipresence.

General practice is not so acutely, devastatingly tiring as working as a houseman, but the steady drip, drip, drip of being on call does take its toll. Until the blessed relief of the co-op, that is, which came into force in our area several years ago. Briefly, instead of each partner in the practice taking it in turns to cover the out of hours commitment to their own patients – in other words, if there are seven of you, you need work only one night a week, while if there are just two of you, it comes to seven nights per fortnight – a co-op consists of a large group of doctors who join together to cover a predetermined geographical area, seeing any patient who may fall ill during their shift irrespective of which practice they belong to.

The individual doctors work shifts of five to seven hours, usually based at a local hospital, and then go home. It is a wonderful system and I applaud wholeheartedly all those who made it possible. Even when on duty you have the benefit of an answer service with a fellow GP screening the calls, and a fully equipped car, with driver included, to accompany you on your forays into the unknown.

We had been sitting in the local hospital on this particular night when the telephone rang. An apologetic GP from the control centre – I've never actually been there, but I imagine it to be akin to the captain's deck on the Starship Enterprise – said:

'I'm terribly sorry, Mike, but I don't think I can put this one off any longer. I've had this wretched woman on the phone four times now, saying her husband is going to commit suicide. It seems they are separated, and when he came home to collect some of his belongings he found her in bed with her new man. Apparently he ran out of the door and disappeared into the night. She hasn't seen sight or sound of him since.'

All very reasonable so far, I thought.

'Trouble is,' he continued, 'this actually happened two weeks ago, and she still hasn't been able to find him. God knows what made her ring tonight, but apparently she's rung the police, who – surprise, surprise – were not all that interested, so now she's ringing us.'

He paused and I could hear him talking to somebody else in the room.

280

'She's on the phone again,' he said, returning. 'I know it's probably going to turn out to be the world's ultimate wild-goose chase, but you know how it is . . .'

I did. It was in the early days of the co-op and already we had had more than our fair share of bad press as the general public began to adjust to taking some of the responsibility for their own health on themselves, poor lambs, rather than depositing it firmly on the shoulders of their doctors.

I could just visualise the headlines.

'Co-op ignores suicide plea.' 'GP refuses to visit dying man'. 'Widow sues doctor after tragic loss.'

We live in a litigation-conscious society, and nobody is more aware of it than ourselves.

'It's OK,' I reassured him. 'We'll miss the last half-hour of the best film I've ever seen and leave the warmth and comfort of our chairs for the bitter night air to do our duty, no matter what the personal cost. It's our job, our vocation, our destiny – '

'Shut up, Mike,' he said good-humouredly. 'Um . . . there is just one other minor difficulty.' He paused.

'Yes?' I said absently, eyes glued on the car chase unfolding on the television before me.

'We don't know precisely where he is. His wife thinks he must be in his caravan . . .'

'Only about five-thousand of those in Widemouth,' I interjected sweetly.

'. . . in a field near a bridge . . . with a broken signpost beside it,' he continued, totally undaunted.

'Oh brilliant!' I said. 'That should be easy to find, then.'

'But we don't actually know which field, or exactly which bridge. Just do the best you can, will you?'

We had been driving now for nearly two hours, and admired virtually every bridge in North Devon and Cornwall, comparing their aesthetic qualities and giving them marks out of ten for degree of hump, inaccessibility and distance from the nearest blind corner.

We had discussed politics, sex, death and the last episode of *Emmerdale Farm*, but what we hadn't done was find our bridge, or our signpost, or our patient.

'Last bridge,' said Colin, the driver, peering through the rain as we drew to a halt. 'And look,' he added, suddenly alert, 'a broken signpost.'

'That's the twelfth broken signpost we've seen tonight,' I reminded him. 'This is North Cornwall, after all. Most of the signposts here are still made out of papier mâché.'

'Go to it, doc,' he said, resolutely ignoring me. 'I'll look after the car. In case . . .'

'. . . there's a message come through on the radio,' I finished for him. 'Don't you worry yourself, Colin. The thought that you will be with me in spirit, as I trudge through yet more muddy fields without a raincoat whilst you sit in a warm, comfortable car listening to the radio, will sustain me tremendously.'

I took the torch, and my bag, and set out in the pelting rain. My last hour's experience of muddy fields had prepared me for almost anything, but this was the muddiest and the worst. I felt thoroughly miserable. It was a hopeless task, and I knew it. I had decided to give up when suddenly, through the drumming of the rain and the howling of the wind, I heard the barking of a dog.

Doctors, postmen and milkmen have one uncanny ability in common. We can all tell from a single bark which dog is tied up and safe, and which is roaming free, all the better to sink its teeth into us.

This dog, irrefutably, was tethered. There wasn't a house for miles around – I had to be in the right place. I followed the sounds through the dark, flashing my torch this way and that and determining to add a pair of wellies to my ever enlarging travelling kit, which already included a thermos flask, a sleeping bag and a complete set of Just William books, and as the barking grew louder I began to contemplate the addition of a shotgun and some tranquillising darts.

And then suddenly I found them – not one dog, but two, possibly the largest Alsatians I have ever seen in my life. They were chained to kennels, one either side of the caravan, their chains long enough to circumnavigate the entire area. I could not get within twenty yards of it.

There was no sign of occupancy within. My prospective patient, if indeed he was inside, was no doubt fast asleep, entirely oblivious to the events outside his retreat. Sleeping, or . . .

I closed my mind to the prospect. What to do next? Calling, or even shouting, was obviously useless. My words would be swept away in an instant by the wind. I couldn't reach the door, there were no stones to throw . . . what could I possibly do? I was just about to give up in despair when inspiration suddenly dawned.

When I was a child – well, OK, when I was a student – I was an avid reader of children's comics. My flatmates and I had delivered to our door each week the *Beano*, *Dandy* and *2000 AD*, not to mention the *Fabulous Furry Freak Brothers*, which we had delivered for an entirely different reason.

One of the comics had a sort of lateral-thinking problem each week. I forget which, but I know it can't possibly have been the *Fabulous Furry Freak Brothers* as thinking – lateral or otherwise – was generally beyond their limited capabilities. This precise problem – well, not involving freezing cold doctors and potentially suicidal patients in caravans in the middle of nowhere in what now was verging on a total blizzard – had appeared in its very pages.

All I needed was a tree.

Cornwall, beautiful, enchanting county though it is, is lacking in many things – indoor toilets, easily understood dialects, roads which actually go somewhere – but it does not lack for trees. There was one only a few yards away.

I approached the nearest Alsatian as close as I dared, who snarled at me, saliva oozing from his wolverine jaws. His chain pulled taut behind him.

Just like a Tom and Jerry cartoon, I thought inconsequentially.

I inched towards the tree. The Alsatian followed, straining every sinew in his body to get at me. Round and round the tree we went, his chain shortening on each circuit until he was well and truly trussed up, and had only a few feet of chain to play with.

There is no such thing as a wasted youth, I thought smugly. After all, biochemistry would never have got me out of this one.

I circumnavigated the other Alsatian and arrived at the caravan door, blessedly out of his reach. Opening it I went inside, wondering what I was to find. My torch picked out a small oil lamp on a tiny kitchen table, with matches beside it, and I lit it carefully.

The inside of the caravan slowly appeared before my eyes. There, in the corner, was a bed, and on it the motionless figure of a middle-aged man in a vest and shorts half covered by a torn and grubby sheet. There were unwashed plates, empty beer cans and over-flowing ashtrays wherever I looked.

Too late, I thought sadly, and walked across to where he lay.

I reached forward and touched the inert body, suddenly to recoil as he sat up with a start and looked at me blearily.

'And who the bloody hell might you be?' he asked belligerently. He saw the stethoscope round my neck and realisation dawned. 'Doctor,' he said, rubbing his eyes wearily. 'Don't tell me – my wife, I suppose. How the hell did you find me?'

His name was Peter, an intelligent, engaging accountant, run to seed. Too many cigarettes, too much whisky, too many problems. In this strange, surreal setting we sat and we talked, sharing a cigarette or two and a tumbler of surprisingly good malt. He opened the door and stepped out in the rain, re-emerging a few seconds later with the two Alsatians, beautiful, pedigree specimens, who lay obediently at his feet, panting heavily.

'My protection,' he explained, 'but they won't harm you, now. If you ever meet them again, they'll treat you as a friend.'

He wasn't suicidal, he said. He was troubled but resigned to his fate, and despite his appearance and setting was a humorous, gentle man, and I warmed to him.

'I'm a diabetic,' he told me at one point. 'On insulin. I could kill myself with a single injection any time I like, as we both know. But I'm not going to do it tonight, doc, so don't worry.'

We talked some more, and then he held out his hand. 'Thanks for coming. I'll be fine, I promise you. Wouldn't dream of doing anything after you've come all this way to see me.' He laughed briefly. 'After all, you still have your career to think of. Can't afford suicides after you've just left a patient on their own, now can you?'

He paused, and his eyes met mine. 'Thanks,' he said. 'I really do appreciate it.'

I walked soberly back to the car, impervious to the driving rain, reflecting on the injustices of the world and how all our lives hang in the balance. There but for the grace of God . . .

I checked my watch. An hour had passed and I started to run, as best I could. Colin would be worried. As I clambered into the car I found him, head back, mouth open, snoring loudly, without a care in the world . . .

There is sadly a footnote to this tale.

Some three months later I bumped into Peter's GP, whom I had not seen for some time, and as we chatted idly of this and that I asked him how Peter was getting on.

He had committed suicide, he told me, from an overdose of insulin about two months after my visit.

I thought of the dogs, those ferociously beautiful beasts, and asked what had happened to them. His wife had had them put down, the following day.

It can be a cruel world sometimes, out there in general practice.

You drift on occasion into people's lives like a piece of flotsam, and then drift away again, unthinking. But their life goes on without you, to its inevitable conclusion, and nothing you can do will ever alter that.

It is a lesson we all have to learn, sooner or later.

But it's not a lesson that ever comes easy.

15

A Sense of Humour

There are a few prerequisites for surviving in this world as a doctor, but only two that are essential. A sense of humour – the blacker the better – and the ability to be totally unfazed by whatever experience should come your way.

Doctors in general, and GPs in particular, are a strange bunch. I do not, of course, include myself in this sweeping generalisation. We spend our lives dealing with other people's miseries, diseases and untimely deaths. Life itself is a terminal disease, and all our patients will one day succumb. We just try and postpone the anticipated date, that's all. So how do we cope?

Well, as mentioned previously, quite simply some of us do not. Depression, divorce, alcoholism, drug addiction, suicide – and that's all before most of us qualify.

The greatest defence of all is the acquisition of that most glorious gift, humour.

But ours is a dark, macabre, black humour, one that many people just do not understand. Seemingly casual, apparently offhand remarks between doctors in often tragic circumstances become almost second nature, and we all recognise this for just what it is – a way of being able to lighten the moment and allow us to deal with the next tragedy, and the one after that, without it taking its toll on us. A depressed, grief-stricken doctor is of no use to his patients.

The trouble is you do sometimes forget that the general public are not quite as inured to such apparent lack of sensitivities as we ourselves . . .

I was sitting quietly at home one evening, watching an old

Western, when the phone rang. I was actually off duty, but when you live in the small village that forms the centre of your practice your home sometimes appears to be public property. An English doctor's home seems doomed never to be his castle.

A breathless voice I did not recognise spoke rapidly. 'We've got a problem over at the school. Quickly, please can you come quickly.' The line went dead.

It was 9.30 p.m. and obviously not a school function. I remembered, in fact, an overheard comment from early in the day about a council or parish meeting, and ambled across the road to see what was going on.

The lights from the school were blazing like a beacon into the cold night air, and I walked through the small, crowded car park into what initially seemed like an empty building.

In rural Devon you never feel uneasy, merely curious. 'Hello,' I called. 'Anyone here?' Silence. I tried again, raising my voice a little. 'Hello?'

A door opened to my left, and I walked through to find a group of the local good and noble gathered around what appeared to be a school curtain on the floor. They were all white, shocked and pallid. As I glanced down at the curtain I realised that it took the shape of the body lying beneath it. At one end, a pair of highly polished brown brogues protruded motionlessly.

'We think he's dead,' spoke one of the gathered throng in a hushed tone, 'but we wanted you to tell us. We didn't know what to do.'

One of the brogues toppled slightly to the left, and my audience gulped and stood back. But I'm a doctor, I could cope. I bent down, pulling the curtain to one side, and there before me lay the recently departed Samuel Parfitt, a warm, kindly man I had known and liked for many years.

He was my next-door neighbour. I groped for the right words. I think the John Wayne film I had been watching must have been foremost in my mind.

287

'Well,' I said, drawling slightly, 'at least he died with his boots on . . .'

But it isn't just ourselves.

It still fascinates me what patients will sometimes say, whereas I am used to the vagaries of doctors' comments regarding those on whom their living sometimes (though to be honest, not all that often) depends.

Indeed my own career was nearly nipped almost before it had begun to bud when, as a student on a ward round, I very accurately but somewhat impolitely described a terminally verbose and consti-pated hospital administrator appositely confined to one of the very wards he administrated as being 'full of shit, both literally and metaphorically'. This came shortly after agreeing that a patient did have rampant diarrhoea, but only of the verbal kind.

I therefore quickly and painfully learned that diplomacy and a desire for some sort of medical future dictated I should cease to be so literally honest, at least in public.

In the good old days, when we were still gods sitting proudly atop our self-erected pedestals, doctors could, and did, write what they liked about patients – be it true, defamatory or purely mischie-vous. I have read, for example 'I examined this patient as thoroughly as I have ever examined any. I could find signs of physical activity, but nowhere could I establish the merest atom of intelligent life. I think you may have referred me an amoeba by mistake.'

Or, 'I assume this patient to be in possession of a functioning cerebral cortex' (brain to you or me) 'as he negotiated the public transport system to arrive here. I was, however, unable to detect its precise location.'

Or then again, 'Another neurone and he'd have a synapse.' (You may need a medical dictionary for this one.)

And even, 'I was so excited by your patient, I thought that at last I had discovered the missing link. It was only when I realised he was still living and breathing I had to sadly conclude that this was not so.'

I must at this point confess to writing – once – 'This man has an irritating complaint. The complaint is in fact less irritating to him than he is to me, and it is for the latter that I have referred him to your good self. He desires his skin to be free of his affliction, whereas I merely require my surgery to be free of mine.'

Oh happy days. Politically incorrect, open to gross misinterpretation and subject to extreme personal bias, I grant you. But doctors could at least communicate their feelings about patients to each other, and share – and of course professionally bond to – our frustrations in dealing with these lesser mortals . . . sorry, the public at large. We can no longer do this, which is of course to the benefit of society, protects individual freedoms and keeps our self-inflated bigotry at bay.

So we just do it by phone instead.

Even now, however, the occasional dark side creeps in. Only recently I received a letter from a chest physician stating, 'I am sorry I cannot give you a definitive diagnosis, as I was most interested in this patient and her lungs. I will be even more interested in them both when she no longer requires them for her own use.'

Interpret that as you wish.

Back to patients.

I went to visit a very deaf elderly lady in one of our local residential homes the other week. We normally have to communicate by blackboard if we want to ask her a specific question, although she can lip read a little.

Her face lit up as I entered the room, which I mistakenly thought was due to her pleasure in seeing me. Not so.

'Have you brought me some of that nice bread?' she asked in eager anticipation.

The matron, once she had stopped giggling, bent down to her ear and bellowed, 'It's the doctor, Mrs Ecclestone, not the baker.' Mrs Ecclestone treated her to a withering glare. 'Yes, I know that, dear,' she said gently, 'but has he got any of those chocolate éclairs I like so much . . . ?'

Worst excuse and most twisted logic for requesting a visit? 'Well, I would have come down to the surgery, doctor, but I was worried I wouldn't be in when you called.'

And then there was the man who insisted his wife was too ill to travel the eight hundred yards to the surgery for an appointment, and yet when I visited responded angrily by saying, 'She was feeling so unwell waiting for you to come that she went into town' (five miles away) 'to do her shopping and take her mind off it.'

Some patients seem to specialise in inverted logic. A middle-aged man whom I had once stopped to help when he had broken down on a deserted country road, was waiting on the doorstep when I visited one morning.

'My car won't start,' he began by way of explanation, 'and I wondered if I could borrow your jump leads again.' I must have looked almost as angry as I was beginning to feel, because he added good-humouredly, 'No, no, it's all right, because I'm not feeling too well and I'd made an appointment to see you to-morrow. Now,' he added virtuously, 'my car will start, and I'll be able to come down and see you and you won't need to visit me after all. You see?'

I did see. It just didn't make me feel any better.

Sometimes you cannot understand what patients are saying at all.

I remember overhearing a long conversation between my receptionist and a local man in his fifties whose accent was so broad it totally defied my interpretation. I was greatly impressed by the way she seemed to understand precisely what he was wanting and dealt with him accordingly. Afterwards – having recently read an article suggesting we should actually talk to our staff, and occasionally even praise them when they have done well – I told her how much I admired her patient interaction skills and asked what the conversation had been about.

'Haven't a clue,' she replied with a shrug. 'I only understood two words. The first one was Tavistock, and the second one Friday.'

The patient has been known to us all as Tavistock Friday ever since, and I have just learned to nod and smile more when faced with an accent I am unable to understand.

Years of training – courtesy of telephone conversations with my mother – have helped, of course. I used to swear that I could answer a call from her, go off, play a round of golf and, picking up the phone again on returning, say, 'Nice to talk to you, but I must be off now,' and she would be none the wiser.

It's not true of course – I need to interject with an 'Oh, really' or 'How interesting' at least every ten minutes, and must use at least one 'How awful for you' and a couple of 'She didn't say that, surely?'

In addition, it helps to have had a father who grunts behind his morning newspaper – grunt interpretation is a must for all aspiring GPs – and, in order to develop a lifelong immunity to social embarrassment, a sister who frequents Etam and Chelsea Girl and wants you to go with her to carry the shopping. If she is also blessed with an ability to spend the entire afternoon trying on clothes and finding nothing she likes, only to return to buy the first thing she saw, then a mere smattering of medical knowledge and you're laughing.

I don't have a brother, and am consequently uncertain what useful function they might provide. Answers on a postcard, please.

I did have a grandmother, however, all four foot eleven of her, who lived to the grand old age of ninety-three despite – though I like to think because of – a lifelong addiction to Park Drive cigarettes. She only stopped smoking when she couldn't see which end to light, and died shortly afterwards, her only residual pleasure in life being finally denied her.

She taught me that deaf people can always hear that which they most covet – whisper the words 'Cherry brandy' within a hundred yards and her eyes would light up instantly – and that just because you can die from smoking does not mean that you have to.

She also used to demonstrate the sheer frustration of her

increasing age and infirmity by walking up to me and punching me with all her might on my upper arm. 'There, I feel better now,' she would say, and potter happily away.

GPs are sometimes there for patients to relieve their frustrations upon too, whether we like it or not. Sometimes it irritates, or angers, and sometimes we understand, but it is part of the job and we should endeavour to see it as such. I tried so hard to understand the man who rammed my car in the surgery car park due to his frustration at my inability to diagnose his long-standing minor ailment and who was purely demonstrating his difficulty in coping with the situation. I tried, I really did.

But I failed, and sued him instead.

Consultations do not always turn out as anticipated. After the recent – and I have to say, totally anticipated – death of a patient, her husband rang and asked if he could come and see me when the surgery was quiet.

Great, I thought. We had, I felt, looked after his wife wonderfully well throughout her long terminal illness, and he was obviously coming to thank us for our hard work, dedication and compassion. GPs love being told how wonderful and caring they are, particularly if there is a bottle of something alcoholic to go with it.

He sat before me and I prepared my 'Oh, we're only too glad to have helped/such a difficult time for you,' speech, to be rounded off with a purely spontaneous 'Oh, you shouldn't have!' as the bottle of eagerly anticipated Chivas Regal landed on my desk.

He looked me squarely in the eye. 'I just wanted to tell you,' he began, and I squirmed a bit. I do get embarrassed with the 'how wonderful you are' part, much as I secretly enjoy it. '. . . that you will be getting a letter from my solicitors tomorrow. Nothing personal, I'm sure you did your best, but I am suing you and the hospital for failing to diagnose my wife's cancer early enough.'

I'm usually ready for most things, but even I was a little taken aback by this. I searched hard for the appropriate phrase to suit the gravity and potential seriousness of the situation.

'So the bottle of Chivas Regal is off then?' I said politely.

I have another patient – one of the 'Oh God, not him again' variety – with several quite debilitating conditions. He is always phoning to explain in the most exhaustive and intimate detail which of his various orifices have been recently explored, how long it took and precisely how painful or thought-provoking it subsequently was. I have often wondered which he enjoys more – having cold bits of metal inserted into unmentionable places or regaling others with the story of the whole enterprise.

Yet whenever he staggers painfully into the surgery to gladden my day with tidings of his trials and tribulations, he ignores the fact that I can actually see, examine, diagnose and occasionally even help. Instead he bewails the administrative trivia that have befallen him on his recent hospital visits.

'Two hours I had to wait for the doctor, and did he apologise? Did he? And then I had to pay £3 each way for the hospital car – *each way* – I ask you, is that fair, and I said to the driver I suppose if you'd been on time it would have been £4, and he was so rude I complained to the ward staff, and they said . . .'

You can see where mothers come in useful.

I am generally a fairly patient man, and if time allows will let the poor unfortunate before me find their own way to the reason for their visit. This is of course unless a test match is on, in which case they are diagnosed, treated and prescribed for as I watch them cross the surgery waiting room – if I'm uncertain, I simply treat them for whatever it was they had the visit before last. You will normally be right eighty per cent of the time.

But Mr Villiers had developed prevarication into an art form. If there was a Turner Prize for it, he would scoop the first three places. The consultation seemed to have lasted all week, and we had discussed everything from how his chilblains were better, thank you, to my recommendations for the best and most hygienic way to trim his ear hair (answer, get someone else to do it) when my patience finally ran out.

It is of course purely coincidental that at that precise moment the afternoon tea break was over and on the television in my consulting room I could see England were walking out to bat at Lords. I would have trimmed Mr Villiers' ear hair myself, and thrown in a shampoo and set as well, just to get him out of the surgery. Time for action. I resolved to be firm, but diplomatic.

'OK, Mr Villiers, I give up, what the bloody hell is wrong with you? Pleasure though it is for you to enjoy the benefit of my company, I have to limit it sooner or later. It's just not fair on all those other people outside who want to waste my time just as much as you do.'

He came to the point – sort of. It was one of those delicious consultations where you just knew the patient absolutely, completely, indisputably, under no circumstances whatsoever wanted to tell you what the problem was, but equally indisputably knew they had to.

Twenty minutes later we finally established that he had a rectal problem. On entering my suitably be-gloved right forefinger into his rectum it was immediately apparent that two things were there that had no right to be. One, of course, was my finger, and the other something hard, solid and completely immovable.

When faced with the unexpected like this, you might think that our immediate concern is for the patient, their welfare and discomfort.

Which is of course completely untrue. What I was really interested in was what it was, how it got there and how good an after-dinner story it would eventually make.

Sadly, I had to wait to find out. Later that day, a surgical registrar rang me and between fits of Brian Johnston-like giggles, interrupted by long spells of silent uncontrollable shaking, he managed to splutter out the truth.

'It was a jar of Coleman's mustard,' he explained. 'Apparently . . .'

– long gap – 'he was walking around the kitchen without any clothes on, and thinks he must have inadvertently sat down on it. He looked at me . . .' There was a silence so long at the other end of the phone I thought he must have dashed off for an emergency appendectomy and a couple of gall bladder removals. '. . . and said, "Do you know, I wondered where that jar of mustard had gone."'

But the best was still to come. 'And then he said, "Lucky the top was still on. At least I didn't waste any . . ."'

The moral of this cautionary tale is never turn your back on a jar of Coleman's mustard, particularly when naked and in the kitchen. They are slippery little devils, and obviously not to be trusted.

The moral of the next tale I leave you to decide on your own.

I was in casualty one day when a man came in wearing an over-coat. Nothing unusual about that, you might think, but this was 1 p.m. on the hottest day in the hottest summer I can recall. Not only that, but where his shoulders should have been – and no doubt actually still were – there was an indefinable something else. Something lumpy and peculiar.

And not only that, either, but he looked a bit strange – and not just because of some extra development in the shoulder department. I know embarrassment when I see it – it's that look you can observe in the mirror after one of those nights, like the one where at the lavish civic ball celebrating the inauguration of your stepfather as the local mayor, you ask the previous mayor's wife if a lady in her position should not by now have developed a better dress sense while your mother is cowering in the corner telling all who are within earshot, 'No, he's not my son, really. He couldn't come and sent a chap he once met on a train as a stand-in.'

I suggested he came to a cubicle and undressed. He hesitated, looking as if cubicles and undressing were the two last things on his mind at present. I took pity on him – well, no, actually that is a lie. I was so intrigued by his as yet undiscovered predicament that I had no intention of letting him leave without him sharing it with me.

'I don't know what your problem is,' I said as sympathetically as I could manage, 'but we see everything here. Nothing surprises or disturbs us, and everything is completely confidential. Trust me, I'm . . .' and I nearly said 'I'm a doctor' but it wouldn't come out without choking, '. . . I'm here to help.'

He opened his mouth to speak, and I'm sure he was probably trying to say, ' I think this might surprise you a bit,' but only a little bleating noise came out. I led him meekly to a cubicle where he took his coat off. Now I understood – well, not exactly everything, but I was completely clear about a. the overcoat, b. the embarrassment and c. the fact that I hadn't seen everything and could be surprised after all.

In the cubicle before me stood a man, but he was not a man entirely alone. In fact, he had brought with him rather a lot of vacuum cleaner and they were currently irredeemably joined at . . . well, for the delicate amongst you, let us just say somewhere near the hip.

The story, as it turned out, was that his wife was away and he obviously had no mistress or even a casual acquaintance to hand. He was, however, blessed with a keen imagination, an innovative mind and some general household appliances. I suppose he had just finished the hoovering, and finding time on his hands, so to speak, he had looked at the Electrolux and wondered, 'What if . . . ?'

I suppose if the Wright Brothers had never said "What if" loudly and often we would be unable to take off on our jumbo to Disneyland, whereas if this chap had never said 'What if' he would now have been at home doing the dusting and preparing to change the duvet cover. Instead of which he was looking at me looking at him and his newly acquired appendage and wondering at which point I would collapse in a heap of uncontrollable giggles.

I could have told him. Any second now.

I mumbled something feeble, asked him to lie on the couch,

promised faithfully I would let no one else into the room, and made my escape. Then I collapsed in the corridor outside casualty and had my thoroughly deserved fit of giggles, and about a week and a half later controlled myself and decided I must do something. So I did.

I rounded up the entire casualty staff, lined them up with a promise of something entirely unmissable, and led them one by one past the cubicle curtain whilst they all peeked in.

Casualty closed down for a while – no, not because there were no patients to treat, or funds suddenly ran dry, but because there wasn't a single member of staff able to function in anything remotely approaching a professional capacity for some time.

A scalpel, a delicate and carefully negotiated procedure – I offered to throw in a circumcision, free of charge, but for some reason or other the poor chap declined – and he was free.

I promised him complete anonymity, and I kept my word. I tore up his casualty card and only he and I know his name. There is no way I am ever going to forget it, even if he does. Of course, I'm not a rich man, and if you should be out there, somewhere, and reading this . . . well, I've always wanted a Mercedes . . .

Policemen often have the same macabre sense of humour as doctors.

I was called out one day to a death on the moors. A sad case – a man in his mid-forties had reported to his friends his intention to take his own life, and then disappeared. After three days of searching they found his car parked in a remote spot on Bodmin moor, and his body a mile away on Roughtor peak.

It was cold, bleak, and a long way uphill. I arrived to find the body lying across a rock, and thought how sad it must have been to spend his last few moments alone in such an isolated spot. There had been a question mark over the circumstances of his death as there were some injuries on his face which had initially been thought to have occurred after he died.

We quickly cleared that up – he had taken an overdose and sat on a rocky ledge, quietly awaiting his end. On finally losing consciousness he had obviously toppled forward and fallen on to the rocks some ten feet below, thus causing his facial wounds.

'We found this,' said one of the policemen, a sergeant, handing me a small vial of fluid. It contained a homoeopathic pick-you-up, and as we stood around the three-day-old corpse I read out the label.

'Rescue remedy,' it was called.

The sergeant looked at me studiously. 'Didn't work, did it?' he said with a deadpan expression on his face.

We do say some things without thinking, which often leaves the casual observer dumbstruck by our apparent complete lack of feeling.

'I'm off to visit Mr Elworthy,' I said to the receptionist one morning. 'He's not all that well, so I might be a while.'

'OK,' she replied. 'You haven't got anyone else for an hour or so, and we'll explain that you might be running a bit late.'

I was back in less than thirty minutes.

'That was quick,' she said, surprised at my early return. 'Is he better then?'

'No, he died last night,' I responded, 'so it didn't take nearly as long as I thought.'

Which was true enough, but to the patients in the waiting room overhearing my offhand remarks it must have seemed a mite uncaring.

I am, in many respects, a shy, retiring man, who avoids at all costs the company of doctors on social occasions. Though I can talk to my gardener about the moral dilemmas of the nation's youth, or why Mike Atherton always looks so constipated, I cannot talk to a GP without them regaling me with the usual tales of their wife, children, mistress or car.

I can, however, be occasionally enticed to attend evening meetings, usually consisting of a talk for an hour or so from an eminent local consultant on a suitably topical subject. The subsequent free meal at an expensive restaurant and unlimited good quality wine are of course of no relevance in my acceptance of the invitation. I go instead in the quest for knowledge and a thirst to further my capabilities, the better to treat my patients.

I do like a good glass of wine. The trouble is, I like two glasses infinitely more than one, and three or four even more than that. By the sixth glass my tongue begins to rule my brain instead of vice versa and I may actually start talking. Occasionally I may talk some sense, and on one particular evening, when I was suitably relaxed, I began to tell the drug rep – a pretty girl, who seemed even prettier each time she ordered another bottle of wine – a poignant story from early in my career.

Gradually the conversation around the table died down, and I became aware that everyone was listening . . .

I was driving back from Belize City, in Central America, to the army camp where I was stationed, in a Land-Rover with two young army medics. The roads were pretty terrible and accidents along the route were legion.

The 'main' road, such as it was, ran alongside the river, a deep, fast flowing, dangerous affair surrounded by many jungled swamps amongst which, in the early hours after a particularly alcoholic night in the bar, we would go alligator hunting with submachine guns . . . but that, fortunately, is another story.

As we rounded the bend, a scene of devastation met our eyes.

Two wrecked cars, the occupants of which were obviously dead, lay strewn across the road. The cause of this, a local rusty, battered and supremely unroadworthy coach, had crashed through the trees lining the river, somersaulted in the air and was lying on its roof, three-quarters submerged beneath the fast-flowing waters. Two terrified locals were sitting on the underside of the coach just above the water-line, screaming hysterically.

There were bodies everywhere, people in the water being swept

to their deaths, people hanging on to the wreckage with desperation in their eyes, and beneath the water-line people still trying to
escape their watery tomb.

In the quiet hours, sometimes, I can still hear the screams. It is
something the like of which I have never seen before, and I pray
will never see again.

The driver stopped the Land-Rover, and we clambered out. In
no time, it seemed, the bank was thronging with locals, inhabitants who had appeared from nowhere. There were no houses, or
huts, or vehicles in sight and yet somehow everyone seemed to
know that a tragedy had occurred.

I cannot swim – a fact that has never worried me before, or
since – but at this moment I felt completely useless. My companions, both good swimmers, immediately stripped off their
clothes and dived into the turbulent waters, oblivious of the risks
to themselves. All you could hear was the rushing of the waters
and the cries of the drowning.

To my surprise, for they were not noted for the love of their
fellow man, the locals were also stripping off their clothes and
diving into the river. I warmed to them. I had misunderstood the
callow, totally self-absorbed nature of their character. I stood on
the bank, ready to help the survivors struggle to shore.

One of the army medics bobbed back into sight, swimming
frantically against the tide, a small child in his grasp. He deposited it on shore, and collapsed exhausted for a moment before
diving back in as I began to give the tiny body mouth to mouth
resuscitation. The other medic appeared too, dragging an elderly
lady in his wake who then lay gasping and spluttering on the bank
beside me.

All around me Belizians were diving into the water, and my
heart went out to them and their natural, unselfish courage. But
then, as I worked on the tiny casualty before me, the awful truth
began to dawn. There were no more casualties being brought to
safety. I could see out of the corner of my eye one of the young

army medics struggling in the water, and glistening brown bodies taking a last breath before sinking down to the stricken coach.

But it wasn't survivors they were after.

A young lad, barely eleven or twelve I guess, emerged glistening from the water beside me, holding a cooking pot triumphantly above his head, chattering and waving it excitedly towards his mother who rushed forward and clasped him enthusiastically in her arms, before pushing him back into the water. Another body emerged, and another, and yet more, each with their trophies.

They weren't diving for survivors. They were diving for salvage. More than a hundred people were drowning in the waters, and while my colleagues were risking their lives to save them their countrymen were looting the wreckage, oblivious to the death and carnage around them. I have never felt so cold, so cynical, so despairing of any faith in human nature . . .

The room was quiet, everyone listening. A lady down at the end of the table, the wife of a GP I knew vaguely, said what they were all thinking.

'So what did you do?' she asked gently. 'It must have been so awful.'

At this point I must apologise, albeit belatedly, to my fellow guests, most of whom have probably never forgiven me. But when in doubt, and too many glasses of wine to the good, you resort to your tried and trusted defence mechanisms, however inappropriate they may be.

The memory of the event had affected me more than I would have expected, and I did not want anyone to see how upset I felt. I looked therefore down the table with the most sober, serious and wounded expression I could muster.

'Well,' I said, straight-faced, 'I jumped into the water, oblivious of my personal safety. I felt I just could not, would not stay uninvolved.' There was a sharp intake of breath all around.

301

'And . . . ?' responded my questioner,

I cringe now, when I think of it.

'And I got myself a new suitcase, and a couple of good pairs of shoes . . .'

There are some days when a sense of humour is maybe not such a good acquisition, after all.

16

From Little Acorns

We all of us, from time to time in general practice, receive requests for unusual, bizarre and sometimes downright unnecessary visits. Sometimes they irritate, sometimes amuse, and sometimes they set off a quite unexpected chain of events.

This particular visit was a combination of all three.

I was not surprised when my receptionist told me that Mr Sanders, a hesitant man in his early eighties, was on the phone. Today, being a Tuesday, I would drive past his front door on my way to one of our branch surgeries, some ten miles away. I would generally drop off his medication *en route* and sometimes, if I had time, stop for a cup of tea and a chat.

Mr Sanders still drove an old Austin Cambridge that had seen many years – most, if not all of them, considerably better ones – and would invariably drive down to the surgery on the rare occasions he needed seeing. It would be unusual for him to request a visit, and I assumed he just wanted to check I had his tablets with me.

I answered the phone and he began to say, 'I don't like to bother you, doctor, but . . .'

I was running late, so interrupted before he could get any further.

'It's quite all right, Mr Sanders, I'll drop in to see you on my way out to branch surgery.'

'No, but . . .' he started to say, but again I would not let him finish.

'It's not a problem for me, honestly,' I reassured him. 'It's quite okay. I'll see you later.'

There was a short silence, and then he said quietly, 'Well, would you mind calling in on the way back instead?' I agreed without giving the matter any further thought.

Branch surgery was quiet, as usual – just a small child with an earache and an elderly lady who wanted to know if she could use her haemorrhoid ointment on the dog as well – and I drove off chuckling to myself, stopping at Mr Sanders' house as I passed.

He answered the door and as he stood there, shuffling hesitantly in his normal manner, I asked how I could help. After much umming and aaahing he finally said, 'Well, it's like this doctor. You see, my car has broken down, and I wondered whether you could give me a lift back into town.'

My dignity was mildly affronted, but he was such a nice old chap my irritation soon settled and I agreed to give him a lift. Another anecdote for the coffers, I thought wryly, and we set off back down the road.

As I drove we started talking, not the usual small talk of my visits but really talking. He spoke about the problems of the lack of public transport, and then for the first time mentioned the chest pain he would experience when walking up the hill from the town centre to the car park. He obviously had significant angina, and must have done so for some time.

'Why have you never told me this before?' I asked.

'Well, you're always so busy, doctor, and it's so nice of you to call in with my pills that I don't like to trouble you. Somehow, though, I felt so relaxed as we were driving along that it seemed as if I could talk about it without feeling I was taking up too much of your time.'

I dropped him off in the town centre, with his reassurance that he would be able to get a lift back without any problem and a promise that we would follow up his angina within the week, and drove away thoughtfully. Was that the impression I gave, I wondered, always too busy to bother?

The next day I was again out in the car on one of my regular visits to a nursing home on the fringes of our practice area, when I passed a young patient of mine hitching a lift. On impulse I stopped to pick him up. It seemed he regularly walked this route on a Wednesday, there being no bus service that came anywhere even close to where he wanted to go.

We also chatted as I drove and he mentioned that – although he was not worried about it – he had noticed a lump in his left testicle a month or so previously. I am sure that had I not given him a lift that day he would never have come to see me about it, or at least not until too late. When I examined him at the surgery the next day it was clear that he had an early testicular tumour, and I referred him for urgent assessment.

The coincidence of these two encounters set me to thinking, and that night I sat with a map of the practice area and considered my various journeys throughout the week. Contrary to what I had expected, instead of having a life of fairly haphazard wanderings led by patient demand I did in fact follow a lot of regular patterns, and almost always drove alone.

There was a germ of an idea here – maybe, during my daily travels, I might have a chance to put something back into the community from which I made my living. We had in the past used local post offices for drug collection points, and utilised the milk lady and a whole variety of willing volunteers to deliver prescriptions where necessary. Perhaps I could expand on that.

There is little in the way of public transport in this part of the world, and after all, there were four spare seats in my car, not to mention seven in my people carrier. I sat up late into the night, planning what I could do . . .

'Travel with your doctor' posters in the surgery, perhaps? 'Consult in the stress-free environment of his car.' No, I thought sadly, that would never do. It would be against the Trade Descriptions Act, for a start, and somebody would be bound to sue.

I thought some more. How about group counselling sessions in the people carrier, I wondered excitedly. I could run some smoking cessation clinics, too, they would be a doddle – drive around all day without any cigarettes in the vehicle and refuse to stop at any garages or village shops. In another flash of inspiration I could visualise 'Walk Yourself Fit' programmes – I would take a group of unsuspecting fatties out into the countryside, miles from civilisation, and dump them there to find their own way home.

I caught myself suddenly. This was getting ridiculous, I must be tired. I climbed the stairs slowly to bed, but the visions would not go away. I could make more of my various journeys through the week, I knew I could. From little acorns who knew what towering oaks might eventually grow?

I finally fell asleep dreaming of a network of luxury coaches criss-crossing the countryside, each with a resident doctor roaming the aisles like an air-stewardess, dispensing laxatives and travel sickness pills with gay abandon. Mobile labour wards, vasectomies while you wait – I was just in the process of ordering my first portable hydrotherapy pool when the phone rang and jerked me back to the cold harsh light of reality.

It was Mrs Brookes, and she sounded terrified.

'It's my husband, doctor, his breathing. It's so terrible – please hurry.'

The Brookes lived in an isolated part of the practice about twenty minutes drive away. They were a tiny couple both in their late seventies, typical of so many in our practice with their stoical acceptance of whatever fate life dealt out to them.

Mrs Brookes, Eileen, was crippled by arthritis, unable to move without the help of her zimmer frame and her husband, Arthur, was her lifeline to the outside world. He was phenomenally fit and healthy, despite his advancing years, and we had always thought she would go first. I prayed I would reach there in time.

I drove out to the cottage as quickly as I could, all thoughts of my new-found intentions instantly forgotten. Eileen had somehow managed to struggle to the front door to let me in, and I rushed through to the living room where I found Arthur sitting in a chair by the fireplace, ashen and gulping in air with a desperation that sent a chill through my bones.

I examined him quickly and it was as I had thought – he had acute heart failure and was deteriorating rapidly in front of my eyes. We so rarely see it these days with the advent of modern treatments, but when I first arrived in Devon it was commonplace; two, maybe three such cases a month. The heart suddenly ceases to beat efficiently and the lungs fill with liquid. Patients start drowning in their own body fluids, and it can be frightening to behold.

It was one of those occasions when auto-pilot takes over. I threw my bag onto a chair, broke open several vials of drugs and injected them into a trembling vein in Arthur's elbow, sitting back for a moment exhausted. There was something I hadn't done . . . my mind raced furiously for a moment and then I leapt to my feet again.

The ambulance – I hadn't rung for an ambulance. Arthur was sitting here in front of me, his life draining away before my eyes, and I hadn't even thought of dialling 999. How could I be so stupid?

I rushed to the phone. Thank God help would be here soon.

But this is Cornwall. The emergency staff are wonderful, but in the middle of the night they are so few on the ground. There was nothing available for an hour and a half, and Arthur would be dead by then, no matter what I might do.

There was just no alternative.

'Arthur,' I said urgently, 'it looks like you're coming with me.'

'Please don't die on me now,' I prayed as I carried him out to the car. He was so light and so trusting. 'We'll be at the hospital soon,' I promised. 'You'll be fine there – we'll get you some oxygen and you'll pick up in no time. I just don't think we can wait for the ambulance. Just don't go to sleep, Arthur, listen to me, please, don't go to sleep.'

I screeched into the hospital car-park and burst through the automatic doors into the reception area.

'What the . . . !' exclaimed the casualty sister, Eleanor, aghast as I braked to a halt inches from the disabled toilet. 'Oh, it's you Mike,' she sighed as recognition dawned. 'So what are you up to this time?'

'I've brought you Arthur,' I explained simply. 'Acute heart failure, and he needs some oxygen now.'

'Right,' she said briskly, pressing the alarm bell. 'Oxygen on the way . . . Christine . . . Peter . . .' she called, 'we need some help here.'

I could hear footsteps advancing down the corridor.

'Everything under control, Mike,' said Eleanor. 'But do you think you could just reverse your car out of the casualty department? It's a little in the way right now.'

I saw Arthur safely onto the ward and then went back out to my car for some rest. There was nothing more I could usefully do for the moment, and the decision regarding Arthur's life or death was in the hands of a greater power than my own.

Five o'clock in the morning I awoke with a start. Arthur – How could I have fallen asleep? I stretched my cramped muscles and made my way back on to the ward.

'Oh look, it's return of the king of the bumper cars,' said Eleanor, grinning broadly. 'Remind me never to get in a car with you at the wheel. Come and see how your patient is doing.'

Arthur was sitting up in bed smiling, looking a different man from the one I had left half an hour earlier. This one was pink and healthy and breathing normally.

'Looks like you got me here just in time,' he said. 'Thanks, Doctor Sparrow, thank you so much. I don't know how I would have managed without you.'

I drove home slowly, calling in on Eileen on the way to give her the good news and then sat in my kitchen watching the dawn break across the valley. Today would be the start of my new campaign. Arthur had been just the stimulus I needed.

I didn't know where it was all going to lead, but there was only one way to find out.

That afternoon I had my car valeted.

If other people were to be travelling with me they wouldn't want to share the passenger seat with the usual collection of broken stethoscopes, empty crisp packets and unexplained body hair.

'Very smart,' pronounced Helen, the district nurse when she arrived the next morning. 'What's all this in aid of, then? I thought the only time your car ever got cleaned was when the body shop had it to beat out yet another of the dents you had put in it.'

I explained the idea I had been formulating and she whistled softly. 'My God, it sounds like you've almost rediscovered your vocation,' she said, impressed. 'How is it going to work?'

'I'm not entirely sure, as yet,' I admitted. 'I've had a few grandiose but impractical ideas, but to be honest I'm just going to start opportunistically – picking up patients I know, making more of an effort to deliver medication to the elderly and isolated when I'm in their area, that sort of thing.'

Helen beamed. 'Well, I think I have your first customer for you,' she said. 'Do you still go out to that nursing home in Halwill on Thursday afternoons?'

'Yes, I do,' I said, wondering what was to come.

'Well, you'll pass close by Cynthia Winters' place, won't you? It's only half a mile out of your way. Could you drop these in there for me – they're her incontinence pads, she ran out yesterday and she's desperate. You know what an awful problem she has, and I won't be able to deliver them until tomorrow. Would you mind?'

'Of course not,' I agreed readily. 'I'd be delighted. I shall be going out there just after lunch as usual.'

It was a beautiful afternoon, and I drove out towards Halwill in high spirits. I was full of enthusiasm – my first 'commission', as it were, and although I did not know at this stage quite what I was going to do in the future I had the greatest of ambitions. Maybe a new community spirit could be engendered in the locality, neighbours looking out for neighbours, perhaps, strangers helping each other along the way, to the benefit of us all.

Half a mile from Cynthia's house I saw her familiar figure waddling painfully down the lane, sweating profusely as she carried a small bag of groceries. Perfect – I could give her a lift home and kill two birds with one stone. I braked and drew up beside her, lowering the passenger window as I did.

And then my eye caught the incontinence pads on the seat beside me. Cynthia had been without any at all for the past two days, she was desperate and we all knew she had a major problem. I glanced up, saw the sweat pouring down her face and shuddered. My car had just been valeted.

I thought of Arthur, and how ill he had been last night. My God, he might have been sick all over the dashboard.

'Lovely day, Cynthia, isn't it?' I called out hastily, and roared off into the distance without her.